Radiation Protection
in the Radiologic and Health Sciences

RADIATION PROTECTION in the Radiologic and Health Sciences

Marilyn E. Noz, Ph.D., and
Gerald Q. Maguire, Jr.

Department of Radiology,
New York University Medical School
Department of Radiological and Health Sciences,
Manhattan College

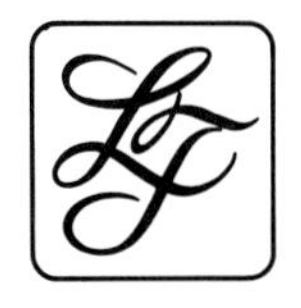

LEA & FEBIGER 1979 Philadelphia

Library of Congress Cataloging in Publication Data

Noz, Marilyn E
Radiation protection in the radiologic and health sciences.

Bibliography: p.
Includes index.
1. Radiation—Safety measures. 2. Radiation dosimetry. I. Maguire, Gerald Q., joint author.
II. Title. [DNLM: 1. Radiation protection. WN650.3 N961r]
RC78.3.N69 1979 614.8'39 78-23698
ISBN 0-8121-0657-1

Published in Great Britain by Henry Kimpton Publishers, London

Printed in the United States of America

Print Number 3 2 1

To our parents and to
Judge and Mrs. Edwin C. Clark

PREFACE

This book would be suitable for courses in an academic or training program in the radiologic and health sciences. It is directed primarily toward students preparing for a career as radiologic technologists or medical health physicists and toward radiology residents. The practicing physician will find it a source of diversified material relating to radiation protection standards and techniques.

As diagnostic and oncologic procedures using ionizing radiation become more and more common, the world has become increasingly concerned about protection of the technician, the physician, the patient, and the innocent bystander who may be exposed to such radiation and thus subject to its harmful effects. Thus, we have decided to produce a readily understandable text on this subject.

For the past 3 years, we have taught the principles of radiation protection in academic and in training programs for technologists, medical health physicists, and radiology residents. Both of us have been extensively involved in the quality control and radiation protection program in the Department of Radiology at the New York University-Bellevue complex.

The book is divided into three sections. The first consists of those principles that have general application; it includes a discussion of instruments used in the field of radiation protection both for area and for personnel monitoring. The proper understanding and use of these principles and instruments are important elements of any radiation protection program. The second section concerns protection from sources of internal radiation. Section three deals with protection from sources of external radiation.

This book includes, as well, four appendices, which outline the basic units of physics, the old units for exposure and absorbed dose, the use of logarithms, along with a table of natural logarithms, and the Greek alphabet. A rather complete glossary of terms is also provided.

The purpose of this book is to provide an understanding of and respect for recommendations relating to the safe use of ionizing radiation in the radiologic and health fields.

As with other such books, this one owes much to the thoughts, criticism, and suggestions of many people, both students and colleagues. We are particularly indebted to Dr. Donald J. Pizzarello for his special help in the preparation of this manuscript and for his encouragement. Our gratitude extends also to Dr. Naomi Harley, James Schimpf, Michael Bonvento, Captain David Alberth, and Carl Mante for their careful reading of the manuscript and many helpful suggestions, and to Georgia Anne Murphy for typing and editorial help. Finally we wish to acknowledge most gratefully the help of Marsha Maguire Roth in preparing the illustrations for publication.

New York

Marilyn E. Noz, Ph.D.
Gerald Q. Maguire, Jr., M.S.

CONTENTS

GENERAL RADIATION PROTECTION

1. Introduction

2. Gas-Filled Detectors

3. Survey Meters

PROTECTION FROM RADIONUCLIDES

8. Good Working Habits

9. Radionuclides and the Law

10. Internal Dosimetry

PROTECTION FROM EXTERNAL RADIATION

11. Barriers

12. External Dose from Photons

APPENDICES

General Radiation Protection

section one

chapter 1

INTRODUCTION

The Food and Drug Administration (FDA) estimates that 130 million Americans have one or more diagnostic x-ray or nuclear medicine examinations annually. The FDA contends that these examinations account for more than 90% of the total man-made radiation exposure to the U.S. population.

NEED FOR RADIATION PROTECTION

One aim of a course in radiation protection for the radiologic and health sciences, then, is to encourage and enable the radiation worker to limit his unnecessary exposure to potentially hazardous radiation. A second and equally important aim is to limit unnecessary exposure to patients and others which results from poor working practices.

The two general classifications of radiation are ionizing and nonionizing. Ionizing radiation is capable of ionizing an atom. Ionization occurs when one of the orbital electrons of an atom has been completely removed from it. The residual atom, which is positively charged, is called a positive ion, or cation; and the freed electron is known as a negative ion, or anion.

That class of radiation able to create ions which are capable of disrupting life processes is known as ionizing radiation. X-rays and beta particles are examples of ionizing radiation. Nonionizing radiation, such as ultraviolet and microwave radiation, lacks the ability to create ions. That such radiation can nevertheless adversely affect human health is a recognized fact. This book is limited to a discussion of protection from ionizing radiation.

Early radiation workers, such as technicians, radiologists, surgeons, and physicists, suffered severe radiation injury because they did not appreciate the extent to which ionizing radiation injures living matter. Further, the development of the nuclear reactor enabled the production of large amounts of artificial radioactivity, which created potential for injury on an unprecedented scale. Many studies have been undertaken to further our understanding of the biologic effects of ionizing radiation and to establish acceptable limits of exposure. Some limited legislation has been enacted with this in mind, and regulatory bodies and licensing mechanisms have been established to set limits for radiation exposure as well as to delineate requirements for training programs for radiation workers. Their aim is to produce a uniformity of accepted practice in working with ionizing radiation.

IONIZING RADIATION AND INJURY

Transfer of energy to the human body may be beneficial, as is the case with food, or injurious, as is the case with a speeding bullet. Ionizing radiation always transfers energy to any material with which it interacts. The energy it deposits in living tissue causes disruption of the atomic structure, and when the atoms thus affected are essential for the normal functioning of a cell, the cell dies. When ionizing radiation imparts energy to living tissue, damage is done: the larger the amount of energy deposited, the more extensive is the damage. Sometimes, for example, in radiation therapy for cancer, this damage can be both beneficial and injurious; it kills the tumorous cells, but it also kills healthy cells.

It is the transferring or depositing of energy in living tissue that is significant in the production of injury by ionizing radiation. As a result all measurements and calculations to evaluate the hazard from ionizing radiation have, as their initial object, the determination of the energy imparted by this radiation to the region of interest.

It has been epidemiologically demonstrated that the damage produced by ionizing radiation is cumulative. An extensive study of the effects of exposure to low levels of radiation over relatively long periods of time was commissioned by the federal government and carried out by the National Academy of Sciences. The results were published in the *BEIR* report (see bibliography).

Three schools of thought exist regarding the effects of exposure to low levels of radiation. In the BEIR report, a linear hypothesis was proposed,

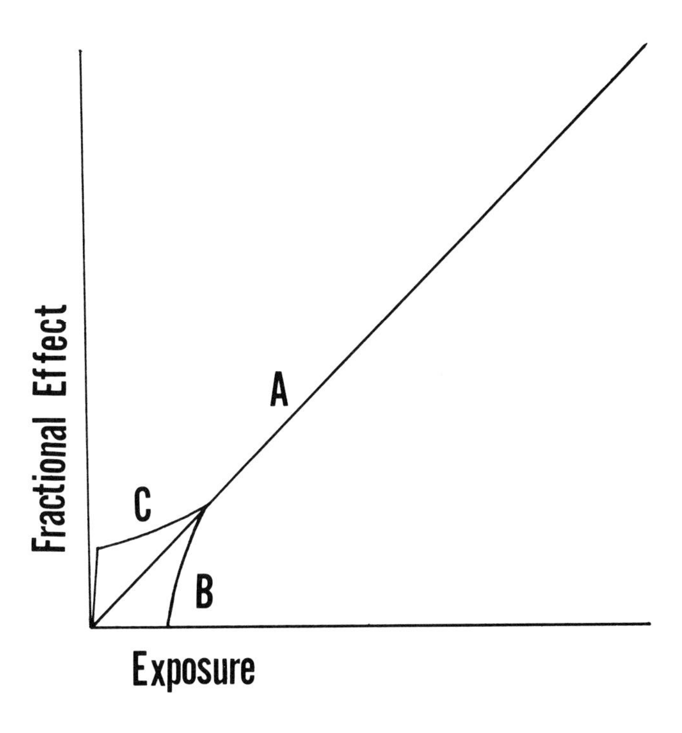

Figure 1.1: Relationship between Radiation Effects and Exposure: Curve A represents the original linear relationship hypothesis. Curve B shows the possible cutoff of radiation effects at low exposure levels (threshold effect). Curve C shows the possible enhancement of radiation effects at low exposure levels.

meaning that the effect was exactly proportional to the amount of exposure (curve A in Fig. 1.1). Later, some researchers felt that a low-limit cutoff for exposure effects may exist (curve B of the same figure). This cutoff is known as the threshold effect. Most recently, some research groups have suggested that effects at low exposure may be more severe than those at higher exposure values (curve C). This controversy is difficult to settle.

Because the body cannot sense exposure to radiation directly, except at levels that are invariably lethal, it can provide no defense against radiation. Hence, it is important to be able to anticipate radiation problems through calculation and analysis. It is equally important to use properly those radiation instruments designed to monitor the emissions from radiation sources.

DIRECT AND INDIRECT IONIZATION

An atom can be ionized in several ways. The method involving ionizing radiation occurs as follows: An electrically charged particle, which has sufficient energy (by virtue of its motion) to release an electron from its orbit, undergoes an inelastic collision with an orbital electron, transferring to it energy at least equal to that of the binding energy of that electron. This transferred energy releases the electron from its orbit.

Thus, ionizing radiation must consist of charged particles, which are capable of ionizing directly, and/or of particles that, though uncharged, are capable of producing charged particles through a secondary mechanism. Electrically charged particles with sufficient energy of motion to produce ionization by collision are called directly ionizing particles. Examples of such particles are electrons, protons, alpha particles, and beta particles. Uncharged particles, which produce ionization only through secondary mechanisms, are known as indirectly ionizing particles. Examples of such particles are photons and neutrons.

ALPHA PARTICLES AND ELECTRONS: DIRECTLY IONIZING PARTICLES

In the health field, two major particles that are charged and, therefore, directly ionizing are alpha particles and electrons. It is important to understand the origin of each of these particles and the way in which each of these behaves in matter.

Alpha Particles

The only natural source of alpha particles is nuclear decay. Some atomic nuclei decay by the expulsion of two neutrons and two protons that are bound together into a particle, commonly known as an alpha particle. These particles are always produced with an energy that is characteristic of the nucleus from which they come. An alpha particle is a helium-4 (^4He) atom with the two electrons stripped away.

Because the alpha particle contains two neutrons and two protons, it has a mass of four units, which makes it an extremely heavy particle. Because it contains two protons, the alpha particle has a charge of +2, which is large and which helps make the alpha particle highly interactive.

The effect of its large mass and its hefty charge makes an alpha particle highly interactive in the vicinity in which it is produced; hence it never penetrates far into any material. A thin sheet of paper is usually sufficient to stop all but the most energetic of alpha particles.

When alpha particles travel through a material, they lose energy by collision with atomic electrons and cause ionization to occur. Their large mass and charge result in a path that is, in general, straight and not very long. The maximum distance that is necessary to stop all alpha particles is known as the range. Even alpha particles with an energy as high as 5 MeV (see Glossary) have a range in tissue of less than 0.04 millimeter.

Electrons

The two major sources of electrons are (1) nuclear decay, in which case they are known as beta particles, and (2) the end product in a material's attenuation of photons having energies in the visible-light region and above. Since neither of these sources produces electrons with a specific energy, in general one is dealing simultaneously with a number of electron energies limited by some maximum energy value. Electrons are very light particles; i.e., they are 2000 times less massive than the proton. The charge on an electron is −1.

Because of its light mass and single charge, an electron is not as interactive as an alpha particle and, therefore, has a much longer range in matter. Also, electrons tend to travel through matter in tortuous paths rather than in straight lines. Usually a few millimeters of aluminum is sufficient to stop the most energetic electrons.

When electrons travel through a material, they lose energy by collision with atomic electrons and thereby cause ionization to occur. Electrons can also lose energy (in the presence of a nucleus) by a braking action, known as bremsstrahlung. In this

Table 1.1

Selected Physical Properties of Some Commonly Used Electrons

Source	^{3}H	^{14}C	^{35}S	^{32}P
Maximum electron energy (MeV)	0.018	0.154	0.167	1.71
Average electron energy (MeV)	0.006	0.050	0.049	0.70
Range in unit-density matter (cm)	0.00052	0.029	0.032	0.8
Fraction transmitted through dead layer of skin (0.007 cm)	0.00	0.11	0.16	0.95

Adapted from Shapiro, J.: Radiation Protection. Cambridge, MA, Harvard University Press, 1972.

instance energy is radiated in the form of a photon, which then produces charged particles (mostly electrons) by the methods described in the next section. Ionization is then caused by the charged particles.

The range of electrons in matter is a function of both the maximum energy of the electrons and the density of the material through which the electrons are travelling. Table 1.1 gives the range for electrons of particular energies in unit density material. Density, symbolized by the greek letter ρ, is defined as mass per unit volume of material. For a unit density material, $\rho=1$. Certain other physical properties of some commonly used electrons are also given in Table 1.1.

It is possible to obtain a relationship between the range R of electrons in a particular material and the density ρ of that material. In fact the range of an electron in a material times the density is equal to a constant number k. In mathematical form:

$$R \cdot \rho = k \tag{1.1}$$

Use of this equation is illustrated in the following example.

Example 1.1

Calculate the minimum thickness of aluminum necessary to stop all the electrons from a phosphorus-32 (^{32}P) source. The maximum electron (beta particle) energy is 1.71 MeV.

From Table 1.1 the range of these electrons in unit density material is 0.8 cm. The density of aluminum is 2.7 g cm^{-3} (cm^3 is commonly written cc). Using equation 1.1 twice,

$$0.8 \text{ cm} \cdot 1 \text{ g cc}^{-1} = k$$

and

$$R \cdot 2.7 \text{ g cc}^{-1} = k$$

Equating the two expressions for k:

$$0.8 \text{ cm} \cdot 1 \text{ g cc}^{-1} = R \cdot 2.7 \text{ g cc}^{-1}$$

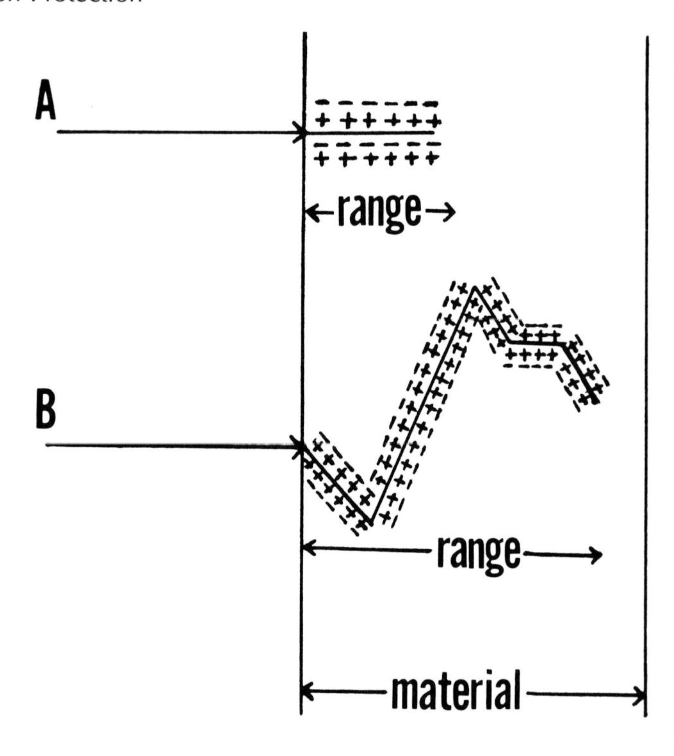

Figure 1.2: Path in matter and range of a 1 MeV alpha particle (A) and an electron (B) of the same energy. Plus and minus signs represent ionization events. (Figure is not to scale.)

Solving for R:

$$R = \frac{0.8 \text{ cm} \cdot 1 \text{ g cc}^{-1}}{2.7 \text{ g cc}^{-1}}$$

$$= 0.3 \text{ cm.}$$

Figure 1.2 illustrates the path and range of alpha particles and electrons traversing matter.

PHOTONS: INDIRECTLY IONIZING PARTICLES

The concept of electromagnetic radiation embraces a large class of physical phenomena: radio and television waves, microwaves, visible light, ultraviolet, x- and gamma radiation. All electromagnetic waves transport energy from one place to another, and this energy travels, or is transported by, the waves in packets or bundles termed quanta. These energy packets give electromagnetic waves their particle-like characteristics. The particle, which characterizes an electromagnetic wave, is called a quantum or photon.

X- and gamma-ray photons are the only types of photons that are of interest in the context of this book, although ultraviolet photons are sometimes used in the radiologic and health sciences. Consequently, the photon energies considered will be between 10 and 5000 keV (0.01 to 5 MeV).

It is important to keep in mind that the difference between x- and gamma-ray photons is in origin, not energy. The term, x-ray photons, is applied to

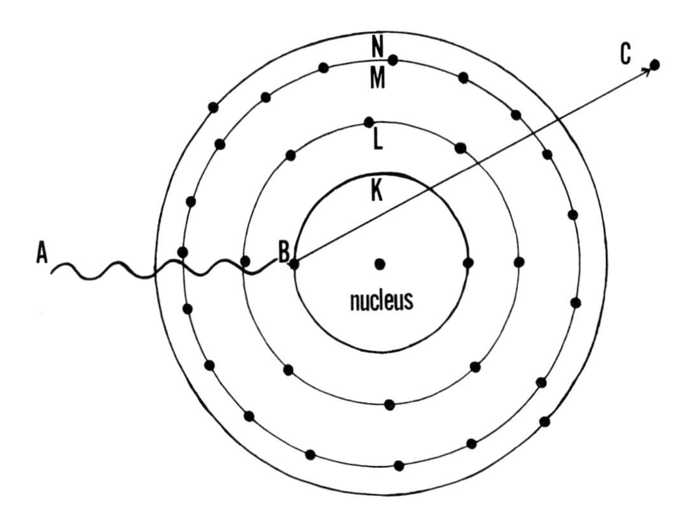

Figure 1.3: The Photoelectric Effect: The incoming photon (A) has an energy equal to or greater than an electron (B) in the K shell. The photon transfers all its energy to the electron, hence releasing the electron from the atom (C). The energy of the electron (C) is equal to the total energy of the photon (A) minus the binding energy of the K shell.

those photons produced by interactions that involve inner-shell electrons in an atom. On the other hand, the term, gamma-ray photon, is applied when photons are the result of interactions involving the atomic nucleus.

Because of the amount of energy associated with them, x- and gamma-ray photons can interact with matter in three special ways. An understanding of each of these interactions is helpful in realizing why x- and gamma-ray photons are potentially harmful, how they are detected in radiation protection work, and why the particular methods used to protect against them are effective.

The first method by which x- and gamma-ray photons interact with matter is known as the photoelectric effect (Fig. 1.3). In this type of interaction a photon has a particle-particle collision with an atomic electron, and the photon transfers all of its energy to the electron. If that energy is sufficient to release the electron from its atomic orbit, the atom is ionized. The freed electron interacts in the manner described in the previous section.

A second way in which x- and gamma-ray photons interact with matter is known as the Compton effect (Fig. 1.4). In this type of interaction a photon collides with an atomic electron. This time, however, it transfers to the electron only part of its energy. The rest of the original photon's energy is radiated as a lower-energy photon. Usually, this secondary photon travels in a different direction from the one creating it. This action is referred to as scattering. It is possible for the lower-energy Compton photon to undergo either a photoelectric or a further Compton interaction. The electron released by the original Compton interaction, and any further electrons released, interact as previously described.

The third method by which x- and gamma-ray photons interact with matter is known as pair production (Fig. 1.5). In this type of interaction the photon, in the presence of a nucleus, disappears, changing all its energy into matter in the form of an electron and a positive electron, known as a positron. In order for this interaction to occur, the photon

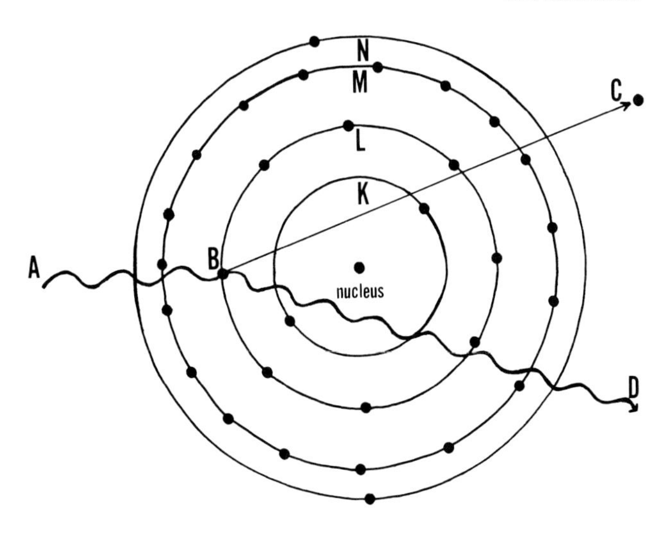

Figure 1.4: The Compton Effect: The incoming photon (A) has an energy much greater than the L-shell binding energy. When the photon (A) interacts with the electron (B), it transfers only some of its energy to the electron. The energy transferred to the electron releases it from the atom (C). The remainder of the photon's (A) energy is re-radiated as a photon (D) of lower energy.

must have an energy of at least 1.02 MeV, i.e., an energy at least equal to the rest mass of the two particles produced (see Glossary). The total energy of the photon is shared equally between the two particles, giving them mass and (perhaps) energy. The electron then interacts as before. The positron loses its extra energy, if any, by ionization. When the positron has lost all its energy, it unites with an electron and the two particles disappear, or annihilate. Two characteristic annihilation gamma photons are produced (Fig. 1–5). These photons each have the same energy—0.511 MeV—and travel in exactly opposite directions. These photons then interact with matter by either the photoelectric or Compton effect.

Although photons do undergo other types of interactions with matter, at the photon energies

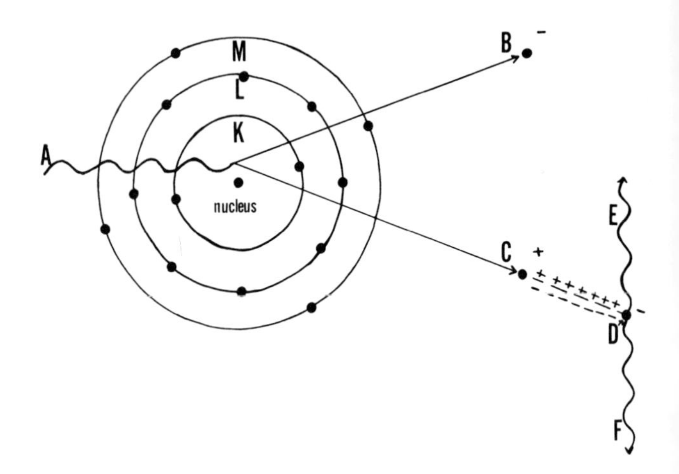

Figure 1.5: Pair Production: A photon (A) of energy greater than 1.02 MeV disintegrates, in the presence of a nucleus, into an electron (B) and a positron (C). The positron loses energy by ionization until it finds an electron (D) and annihilates, producing two characteristic annihilation photons (E and F). Note that the annihilation photons travel in directions exactly opposite to each other.

encountered in the radiologic and health sciences, the three interactions just discussed are the most important ones. Which type of interaction a photon will undergo is determined by two factors: the energy of the photon and the material it is traversing. In general, photons of lower energy (less than 100 keV) are more likely to interact through the photoelectric effect; photons of intermediate energy (100 keV to 1000 keV), through the Compton effect; and photons of energies greater than 1.02 MeV, through pair production. The specific energy range of each interaction is determined by the properties of the material through which the photon is travelling.

Whenever a beam of photons traverses a material, some of the photons interact with the material and are lost from the beam. This process is referred to as attenuation. To attenuate a photon beam means simply to remove some of the photons from it by interactions between the photons and the material. When a photoelectric interaction occurs, all of the photon's energy is absorbed or attenuated out of the beam. When a Compton interaction occurs, some of the photon's energy is absorbed out of the beam and the rest is scattered from the beam by the secondary photon produced.

RADIOACTIVITY

The most common source of alpha and beta particles and of gamma-ray photons is the natural or induced transformation or decay of the nucleus of an atom. Every chemical element has associated with it an atom that has a fixed number of protons in its nucleus and the same number of electrons orbiting about the nucleus. However, the number of neutrons present in the nucleus may vary (and often does). One example is oxygen. The common form of naturally occurring oxygen has eight protons and eight neutrons in the nucleus. However, oxygen also is a stable atom if it has nine or ten neutrons in its nucleus. At the same time, oxygen has another form (with seven neutrons in the nucleus) which decays spontaneously, emitting a positive electron, or positron.

It is common to speak of different nuclear forms as nuclides. When this nuclear form changes, or decays, either by emitting excess energy in the form of a photon or by emitting a particle, or both, the nuclide is referred to as a radionuclide and is said to be radioactive.

Some radionuclides exist in nature; common examples are uranium-238 (^{238}U) and potassium-40 (^{40}K). Other nuclides are made radioactive. For example, tellurium-124 (^{124}Te) can be used as the target material in a cyclotron. When this nuclide absorbs a high-energy proton produced in the cyclotron, it forms iodine-123 (^{123}I) plus two neutrons. ^{123}I then decays spontaneously emitting a photon. The

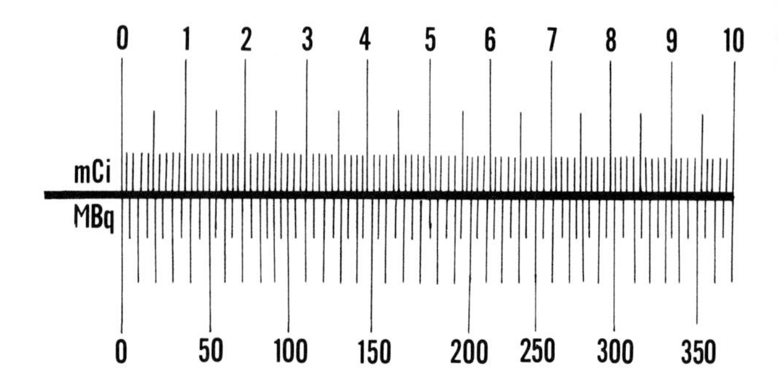

Figure 1.6: Nomogram (conversion scale) showing the conversion from mCi to MBq. (Reprinted with permission from the pamphlet "Units for the Measurement of Radioactivity and Ionizing Radiation" issued by the Metric Conversion Board of Australia, Crow's Nest, NSW, 1977.)

various radioactive decay processes are too extensive to be discussed here (Lederer, 1967).

Each time a radionuclide undergoes a transformation or decay, a new nuclide is produced and is usually accompanied by other decay product(s). These decay products are usually, but not always, an alpha or beta particle and/or a photon. The rate at which radionuclides in a given sample undergo transformations, and, consequently, the rate of emission of the decay product(s), are directly proportional to the number of radioactive nuclides contained therein. Thus as the number of radioactive nuclides in the sample or source decreases because of the radioactive decay taking place, the rate of emission of the decay product(s) also decreases. The rate of emission of the decay product(s) is known as the activity of the source.

In the newly adopted system of measurement, the International System or SI, the unit of radioactivity is the becquerel* (Bq). It is equal to one disintegration, or decay, per second. In the old system of measurement, the unit of radioactivity is the curie* (Ci), which is defined as $3.7 \cdot 10^{10}$ disintegrations per second. Since the curie represents a very large number of disintegrations, it is common to express activities as mCi (one thousandth of a curie), or as μCi (one millionth of a curie). Figure 1.6 gives a simple nomogram or conversion scale between becquerels and curies. Appendix I gives an overview of commonly used systems of measurements.

BIBLIOGRAPHY

The Effects on Populations of Exposure to Low Levels of Ionizing Radiation. Report of the Advisory Committee on the Biological Effects of Ionizing Radiation (BEIR Report). Washington, D.C., Division of Medical Sciences, National Academy of Sciences, National Research Council, 1972 and 1977.

Lederer, C. M., Hollander, J. M., and Perlman, I.: Table of Isotopes, 6th ed. New York, John Wiley & Sons, 1967.

Pizzarello, D. J., and Witcofski, R. L.: Basic Radiation Biology, 2nd ed. Philadelphia, Lea & Febiger, 1975.

Progress in Radiation Protection (U.S. Department of Health, Education and Welfare Publication, FDA No. 77–8015). Rockville, MD, Bureau of Radiological Health, 1975.

*Both the becquerel and the curie are named after scientists who did pioneering work in the field of radioactivity. Henri Becquerel (1852–1908), a French physicist, discovered gamma-ray photons in 1896. Madame Marie Curie (1867–1934), working in France, although she was of Polish birth, discovered artificial radioactivity. Becquerel, Marie Curie and her husband Pierre (1850–1906) received the Nobel prize in physics in 1903 for their work in radioactivity.

chapter 2

Gas-Filled Detectors

Every radiation detection system consists of two parts. The first is the detector proper, where the interaction of radiation and matter takes place. The second is the measuring apparatus, sometimes called the counter or readout component. This takes whatever the detector produces and performs those functions required to accomplish the desired measurements.

Different types of systems are characterized by the nature of the interaction of radiation with the detector. Several types operate by virtue of the ionization produced in the detector by the passage of charged particles. Examples of such systems are ionization chambers, proportional counters, Geiger counters, semiconductor radiation detectors, and cloud and spark chambers.

In these detectors, if the primary radiation consists of charged particles, ionization is produced directly. If the primary radiation consists of uncharged particles, i.e., neutrons or photons, production of ionization originates by secondary processes, as explained in Chapter 1. In the radiologic and health sciences the main thrust is the detection of and protection from photons and (usually fast) beta particles (electrons).

Detection systems, as a whole, are classified by their mode of operation, i.e., whether they are pulse-type or mean-level devices. In the pulse-type mode of operation, the output of the detector is a series of signals, or pulses, resolved or separated in time.

Each signal represents the interaction of a nuclear particle with the detector. A Geiger counter is an example of a detection system that operates in the pulse mode.

In the mean-level or integrating mode of operation, the quantity measured directly is the average effect due to many interactions of radiation with the detector. No attempt is made to resolve individual particles, as such resolution is often impossible because of the high rate at which they occur. An ionization chamber is an example of a detection system that is most often operated in the mean-level mode.

Those systems in which detectors operate by virtue of charged particles producing ionization in a gas-filled chamber are known as gas-filled detectors. The three most common systems of this type are ionization chambers, proportional counters, and Geiger counters.

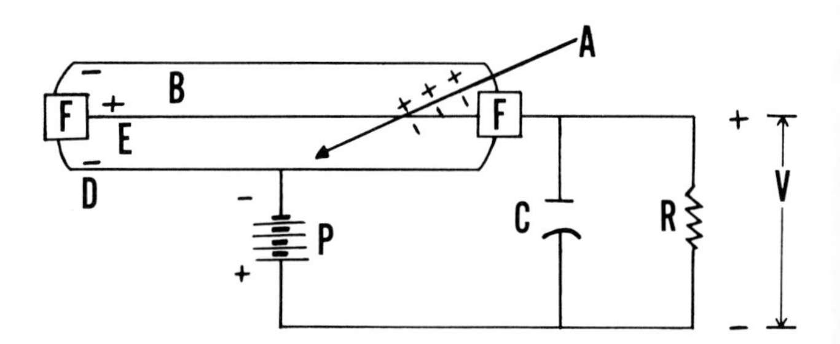

Figure 2.1: A Gas-Filled Detector: The incoming ionizing radiation (A) enters the detector (B) and causes ionization. The residual positive ions move toward the chamber walls (D), which are negatively charged, thus forming the cathode. The electrons (negative ions) move toward the central wire (E), which is positively charged and thus forms the anode. The central wire and the chamber walls are electrically isolated from each other by the insulating material (F). The voltage level (V) is maintained by the power source (P). The resistor (R) capacitor (C) circuit integrates individual pulses from the electrons.

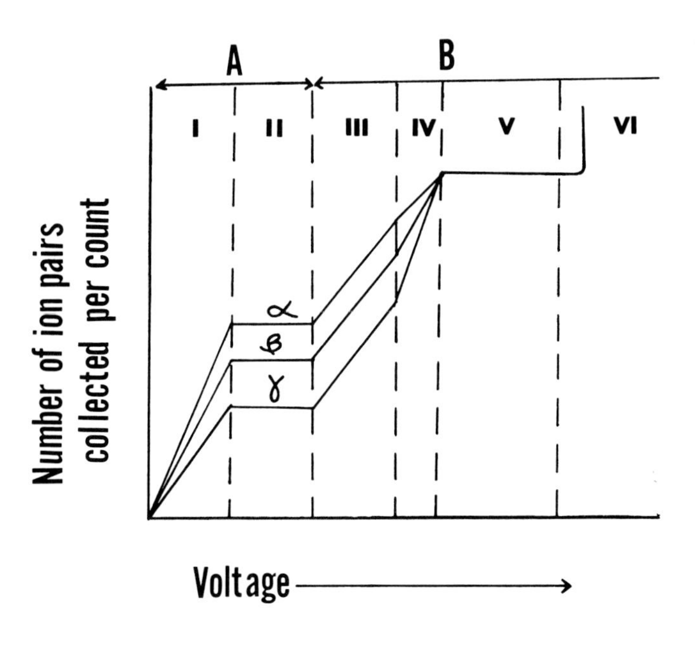

Figure 2.2: Voltage Dependence of a Gas-Filled Detector: Region I represents the voltage levels at which partial recombination of ion pairs take place. Region II is the ionization chamber region. No recombination of ion pairs takes place here, and no secondary electrons are produced. Region III is the region of proportionality. The number of secondary ion pairs produced is directly proportional to the number of primary ion pairs produced. Region IV is the region of limited proportionality. Region V is the Geiger region. Here the maximum number of ion pairs is produced by even one primary ion pair. Region VI is the region of continuous discharge. A represents voltage levels that produce simple ionization. For the voltage levels B, multiplication of primary ionization takes place. (Adapted from Arena, V.: Ionizing Radiation and Life: an introduction to radiation biology and biological radiotracer methods. St. Louis, The C. V. Mosby Co., 1971.)

Detectors associated with each of these systems employ a gas-filled chamber with a positively charged central electrode insulated from the negatively charged chamber walls. A voltage (V), applied between the wall and central electrode, maintains the charge distribution (Fig. 2.1).

The passage of a charged particle through the gas releases ion pairs within the chamber, an ion pair being an atom with a residual positive charge and a negatively charged electron. The positive and negative charge thus produced have a force applied to them by the voltage; positive charges tend to move toward the chamber walls and negative charges toward the central electrode, because opposite charges attract.

The main differences among the three types of gas-filled detectors lie in the gas used, the pressure at which that gas is maintained within the chamber, and the voltage level that is maintained between the central electrode and walls of the chamber. Figure 2.2 is a graph of the voltage versus the amount of ionization that occurs.

The gas-filled detector system known as a proportional counter is used primarily for alpha particles, very low energy electrons, and neutrons. Since, in medical protection work, sources of these particles are rarely encountered, the proportional counter has not been discussed.

THE IONIZATION CHAMBER

Ionization chambers are used as survey meters, as dose calibrators, as personnel monitors, and as standard measuring devices for determining radiation levels. They are useful because they can indicate the quantity of the incoming radiation and in some cases its energy as well. This capability enables the user to identify the source, or radionuclide, as well as the strength of radiation present.

The detector proper can take many forms. The most common is that of a cylindrical conducting chamber containing a central electrode located on the axis of the chamber and insulated from it (see Fig. 2.1).

The usual gas filling for an ionization-chamber detector is dry air at atmospheric pressure, which is equivalent to 760 torr or 760 mm Hg. Other gases are sometimes used for particular purposes, but in medical radiation protection work, air is commonly used.

An ionization chamber can be used to some extent for detection of all types of particles. However, in medical protection work it is most commonly used in the mean-level mode of operation for detection of both photons and high-speed electrons.

The ionization chamber can be used in two ways: (1) as a current-measuring device yielding a quantity proportional to the rate (amount/unit time) of arrival of the ionizing radiation within the detector, and (2) as a voltage-measuring device yielding a quantity related to total radiation incident on the chamber during the entire period of measurement.

Theory of Operation

An ionization chamber demands that only ionization produced directly by incoming radiation be collected. Therefore, for quantitative measurements, the detector must furnish an output having a definite relationship to this ionization. To accomplish this goal, a known fraction of the charge produced within the chamber must be collected and no other ionization can take place. Therefore, it is necessary to understand how the electron and residual positive ions, once formed, behave.

When an outer-shell or valence electron is released from an atom, the immediate inclination of electron and positive ion is to reunite. To avoid this "recombination," a certain minimum level of voltage must be maintained in the ionization chamber. This voltage must exert enough force on the electron to separate it from the positive ion and to send both of them on their respective ways. It is most usual for the walls of the chamber to be the cathode; i.e., they have a negative potential or an excess of electrons. Thus the positive ions, travelling slowly because they are relatively massive, migrate to the chamber walls, where they receive an electron and are neutral once again.

The central wire is usually the anode, which is positive with respect to the chamber walls; hence electrons are attracted to it. Electrons, however, are very light, and a small force applied to them (by the voltage V in the detector) gives them a lot of energy. Therefore, the voltage applied in the chamber must be low enough to keep the electrons from acquiring so much energy before reaching the anode that they (the electrons themselves) ionize other atoms. This type of ionization is called secondary ionization. Usually ionization chambers have voltages between 100 and 300 V, although some have higher operating voltages.

Electron Movement to Electrode

It is illuminating to describe how electrons, once formed, move through the surrounding gas atoms to the electrode. When an electron travels toward the anode, it does so by a crooked path because it collides with the neutral atoms located everywhere in the chamber. The more atoms with which an electron can collide, the more it will do so, and the shorter will be the distance that the electron travels between collisions; also the electron will acquire less energy between collisions. Keep in mind that the voltage applies a force to the electrons, thus giving them energy.

The average distance that an electron travels between collisions is called the mean free path, which is inversely proportional to the pressure of the gas, i.e., to the number of gas molecules per unit volume. When an electron collides with a gas molecule, it is deflected from its original path. The direction of the electron's motion is random; however, the net drift of the negative electron is toward the positive anode. The speed with which the electron drifts toward the anode is known as the drift velocity; it is directly proportional to the applied voltage in the chamber and inversely proportional to the pressure.

One more property of electrons must be taken into account. Electrons have a tendency to attach themselves to neutral atoms, thus forming negative ions. These negative ions are massive and slow and do not drift toward the anode at the same rate as the electrons. Therefore, this property of electrons must be combatted by using a gas whose atoms have a low electron affinity, i.e., do not attach electrons to themselves very readily. The inert gases such as helium, argon, neon, and krypton have a low electron affinity.

The use of ionization chambers as survey meters and personnel monitors is discussed in Chapters 3 and 4.

GEIGER COUNTERS

Geiger counters, also called Geiger-Müller or G-M tubes, are widely used as monitoring instruments because they can detect any type of radiation that produces ionization within the detector, no matter how small the amount of ionization. In fact, this high sensitivity makes Geiger counters ideally suited for detecting fast electrons and photons because the small ionization of these particles would be hard to detect otherwise. Alpha particles and other highly ionizing particles can be detected by G-M tubes, but because of their short range they are unable to penetrate the walls of the detector unless thin windows are used or the source of the radiation is placed inside the detector.

Geiger counters are almost always used in pulse mode. Their theory of operation requires that the number of electrons collected at the anode be independent of the amount of primary ionization. Hence this factor cannot be used as a measure of particle energy, nor is it possible to discriminate among different types of particles by means of the sensitivity of the electronic circuit. Therefore, G-M tubes can tell nothing about the energy of radiation.

The great utility of the G-M tube is the result of several factors:

1. It has very high sensitivity.
2. It can be used with different types of radiation.
3. It can be fabricated in a wide variety of shapes; i.e., the width can be anywhere from 2 mm to several centimeters, and the length, 1 cm to several meters.
4. Its output signal is so strong that it requires little or no amplification.
5. It is reasonable in cost, because the tube, as well as the electronics following it, are extremely simple in construction.

Description

The tube itself is generally a metallic envelope in which two electrodes and a proper filling gas are incorporated. The internal, or collector, electrode (anode) is a fine wire (about $^1/_{10}$ mm in diameter) frequently made of tungsten because of its strength and uniformity in small-diameter wires. The anode is most often supported at both ends with insulators (see Figure 2.1). Sometimes, however, the anode is terminated at one end by a glass bead or a loop. As opposed to the ionization chambers, the most common filling gas for a Geiger counter is one of the noble gases: helium, argon, or neon. The only requirement is that the gas have a small electron affinity. A large range of pressures is used, the most frequent being 70 to 200 torr (millimeters of mercury).

In order to achieve the high sensitivity of the G-M tube, a relatively high operating voltage must be used (generally between 900 and 1200 V). Again this feature differs from that of the ionization chamber.

The quality of a G-M tube is determined by the counting rate versus voltage response, as shown in Figure 2.3. That range of operating voltages through which the counting rate changes very little is called the plateau. A good tube has a counting-rate change of less than 10% throughout the plateau region. The

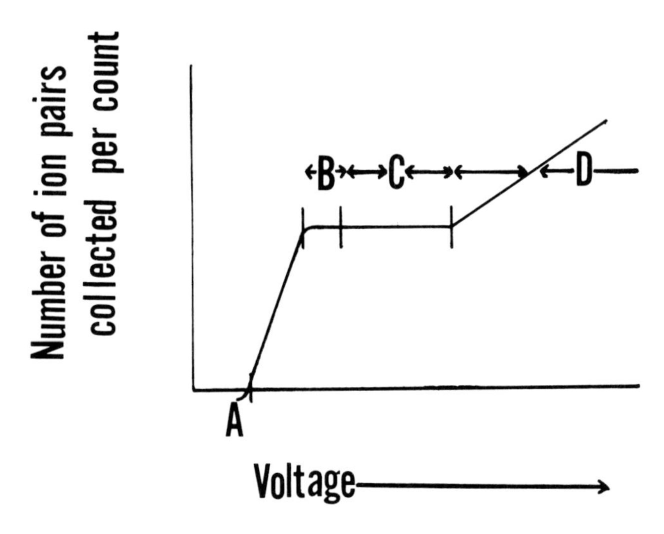

Figure 2.3: Geiger Counter Plateau: A represents the starting potential or starting voltage, B represents the "knee" or threshold voltage, C represents the plateau region, and D represents the breakdown or continuous discharge region.

voltage at which the G-M tube begins to count is known as the starting voltage. Voltages higher than the plateau voltage result in a breakdown of the tube gas; i.e., ionization occurs because the voltage itself pulls the gas atoms apart even without the presence of any ionizing radiation.

Count Method

The production of counts in a G-M tube occurs in the following manner: Electrons produced by the primary ionizing event drift toward the anode but lose energy when they are scattered away from it. The electrons do not gain enough energy between collisions to produce secondary ionization until they arrive within the last few mean free paths of the anode. Once ionization starts, it builds up rapidly, since secondary ionization events can produce more ionization. This buildup is known as a Townsend avalanche (Fig. 2.4).

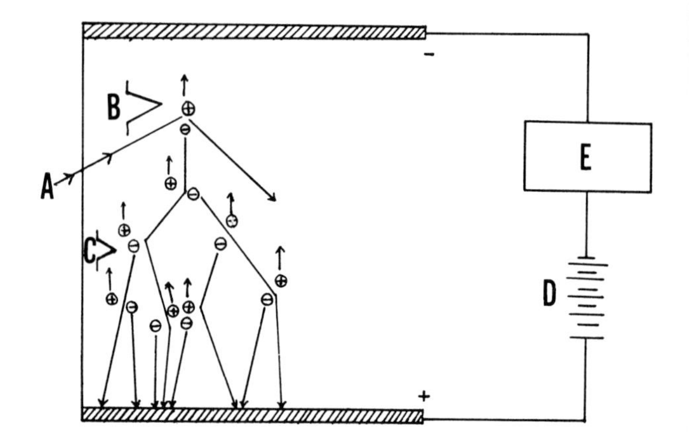

Figure 2.4: Production of Avalanches in a Geiger-Müller Tube: The incoming ionizing radiation (A) forms a primary ion pair (B). The electron thus released produces many secondary ion pairs (C). A very high potential difference or voltage (D) is applied to the tube, and the ionizing events are recorded by the measuring apparatus (E). (Adapted from Arena, V.: Ionizing Radiation and Life: an introduction to radiation biology and biological radiotracer methods. St. Louis, The C. V. Mosby Co., 1971; Courtesy Atomic Energy Commission.)

The initial Townsend avalanche terminates when all the electrons associated with it have reached the anode. However, the initial avalanche is followed by a succession of avalanches, each of which is triggered by the preceding one. The termination of the avalanches comes when the number of positive ions surrounding the anode reduces the voltage of the anode to a level that is inadequate for maintaining ionization.

The entire production of avalanches occurs in a fraction of a microsecond. In this short time electrons are collected at the anode; then the positive ions migrate to the cathode.

It must be kept in mind that the voltage across the G-M tube is high; hence the positive ions are able to gain a lot of energy on their way to the cathode. The collision of these energetic positive ions with the cathode causes either of two effects:

1. An electron is ejected from the cathode with an amount of energy that is the difference between the energy of the positive ion and the ionization potential (work function) of the atoms composing the walls of the cathode. When the electron binds to the positive ion, this energy difference plus the binding energy is radiated as a low-energy photon, which subsequently produces a photoelectron.
2. More than one electron can be ejected directly from the cathode by a single positive ion.

In either case, these "extra" electrons start another series of avalanches if they are not stopped. The procedure used to prevent positive ions from producing further avalanching is called "quenching." Three methods exist for quenching a G-M tube.

Quenching

The first method is known as electronic quenching. In this situation, once avalanching at the anode is stopped, the voltage across the tube itself is lowered. Thus the positive ions do not gain a sufficient amount of kinetic energy to produce excess electrons or photoelectrons. However, this very old method of quenching has the disadvantage that, because of the lowered voltage, positive ions take longer to get to the cathode, so a longer time elapses before the tube is ready to accept another count. Also the electronics connected with the tube must be more complicated, thus raising the cost of the Geiger counter as a whole.

The second method is known as organic quenching. Here, a small amount (about 10%) of organic gas is mixed with ordinary tube gas. Although any alcohol gas will do, common organic gases used are ethanol and ethyl formate. The positive ions, on their way to the cathode, bump into these large, electron-rich organic molecules and transfer their charge to them. The organic molecules, being massive and hence slow, migrate to the cathode and release electrons. The extra energy released in the form of photons or electrons, however, goes to dissociating the organic molecules rather than to starting new avalanches. When all the quenching gas has been dissociated, the G-M tube is no longer quenched and hence no longer useful. Approximately, 10^9 organic molecules are dissociated in each set of avalanches, so an organic quenched G-M tube has a finite lifetime of about 10^{10} counts. Because of its finite lifetime, this method of quenching is infrequently used.

The third method is known as halogen quenching. With this procedure, about 0.1% halogen gas, usually chlorine or bromine, is added to the tube gas. The halogens readily give up an electron to neutralize the positive ions. When the halogen gas gets to the cathode, the extra energy released goes into dissociating the halogen molecule. However, halogen atoms quickly reassociate. Thus the lifetime of the G-M tube that is halogen-quenched is practically infinite. Also it is possible to run the tube at a higher voltage. One precaution must be observed with halogen quenching: The material composing the walls of the tube must not absorb the halogen used.

The sensitive volume of the tube is that volume in which, when a primary ionizing event occurs, an avalanche will result. Halogen-quenched tubes have a larger sensitive volume than, for example, organic quenched tubes.

Resolving Time

Since the G-M tube is a pulse-type device, its resolving time, i.e., the time between counts, must be discussed. The only restriction on the counting system is that it register an avalanching sequence when it occurs in the tube. Once a primary ionizing event starts a series of avalanches, a new primary ionizing event is not detected until the avalanching stops and the positive ions are neutralized.

The dead time is defined as the time from entry of an initial ionizing event until avalanching at the anode terminates; the recovery time, as the time required for complete recovery of the electronics after the end of the dead-time interval; and the resolving time, as the sum of dead time plus recovery time. A good Geiger counter has an electronic circuit that gives a resolving time very close to the dead time. The dead time varies from count to count even in the same G-M tube, but it is typically 100 to 200 μsec. The use of a Geiger counter as a laboratory survey monitor is discussed in Chapter 3.

BIBLIOGRAPHY

Price, W. J.: Survey of detection methods (Chapter 2), ionization chambers (Chapter 4), and the Geiger-Müller counter (Chapter 5). *In* Nuclear Radiation Detection, 2nd ed. New York, McGraw-Hill Book Co., 1964.

chapter 3

SURVEY METERS

The most important use of those gas-filled detectors described in Chapter 2 is as radiation monitoring devices. As a result, they are also known as survey meters or instruments or laboratory monitors. Geiger counters are used as survey instruments while ionization chambers are used for both laboratory and personnel monitoring.

The purpose of a laboratory monitor or survey instrument is twofold: to keep a constant surveillance over the working environment and to detect the quantity and extent of contamination. Consequently, laboratory monitors are placed in rooms where radionuclides are used. Counters, floors, and other places where spills may have occurred are surveyed daily. In addition, rooms containing diagnostic or therapeutic x-ray equipment or other sources of radiation are surveyed periodically for amount of leakage and scattered radiation.

CHARACTERISTICS OF AN EFFECTIVE SURVEY METER

Laboratory survey instruments must possess the following characteristics: simplicity of construction, ruggedness, reliability, portability, and sensitivity.

An instrument that is simply constructed is easy to use. Moreover, its circuitry should be easy to comprehend, its parts readily replaceable, and its components conveniently arranged. These features also enable the survey instrument to be reasonably priced.

A survey instrument must be able to withstand hard use. Since it will most likely be handled by many different people, a survey instrument should be rugged enough to survive mild abuse.

Reliability is another important quality of a survey meter. As is discussed later in this chapter, survey meters, particularly G-M tubes, must be calibrated regularly. In order to ensure that the reading obtained on the meter is a correct one, a small source of radiation (known as a check source) is provided with the meter. When the detector is placed near the check source, a precalibrated reading should be obtained. This procedure should be done immediately prior to use since one of the major functions of a survey meter is to provide an accurate estimate of the amount of radiation present.

Portability is desirable because it is often necessary to use a given survey instrument in a number of different locations. For this reason, the survey meter should be light and compact and should contain its own battery.

Finally, the main reason why a survey meter is present in the area is to monitor contamination or leakage of radiation; consequently, it must be very sensitive to both the type of radiation being monitored and its energy range. For example, in most instances in the radiologic and health sciences, it is necessary to detect photons with energies between 10 and 1000 keV. Hence a Geiger-Müller tube detector or an ionization chamber is usually used. On the other hand, if alpha particles are to be detected, a proportional counter should be used. G-M tubes make excellent monitors because of their high sensitivity to photons in the energy range being considered.

Generally speaking, no one survey instrument will have all of the characteristics described, so it is important to select the proper instrument for a particular monitoring situation. Further, it is necessary to know how to use that instrument intelligently and to be able to interpret the results.

ENERGY DEPENDENCE

Most survey instruments encountered in the radiologic and health sciences are gas-filled detectors. Instruments of this type operate by virtue of the ionization produced in the gas by the radiation to be detected. In general, the meter gives a reading, usually in counts per minute, designed to be an indication of how much radiation is present. Gas-filled detectors have poor energy-dependence characteristics; i.e., their readings depend upon not only the amount of radiation present but also the energy of that radiation. Instruments with good energy dependence characteristics give readings based on the amount of radiation present only and are not influenced by the energy of that radiation.

Energy dependence occurs for two reasons. The first has to do with the material used to make the walls of the detector. By convention, the amount of radiation present is determined by measuring the ionization of air. Consequently, the walls of the chamber in which photons are attenuated should be made of an air-equivalent material, i.e., a material which has the same or nearly the same atomic number (Z) as air. (The Z for air is approximately 7.64.) At the same time, the thickness of the walls is a second factor to be considered. The amount of interaction of photons with the material composing the detector walls, and the penetrating ability of particles emitted are functions of energy. (Recall, from Chapter 1, the methods by which photons interact with matter.) Very high-energy photons have a small interaction probability; i.e., they tend to interact less than lower energy photons; hence the walls of the chamber should be thick. On the other hand, very low-energy photons produce particles that, because of their small penetrating power, do not reach the gas-filling to be detected if the chamber walls are too thick. Hence the thickness of the chamber walls has an effect on the number of photons detected. Ideally, a survey instrument with adjustable walls is best for learning about the energy composition of the radiation.

IONIZATION CHAMBER MONITORS

Ionization chambers can be constructed so as to be useful for any kind of radiation monitoring. They are best used as photon measuring instruments, but they can be modified to monitor for alpha, beta, and even neutron radiations. Furthermore, although ion chambers have less sensitivity than Geiger counters, they can be used in high counting-rate situations, where they give precise results. Since ion chambers have good energy-dependence characteristics, they are desirable instruments for general radiation-safety and survey work.

Ionization chambers, when used for radiation survey work, always operate in the mean-level mode. Energy absorbed from the radiation ionizes the gas in the chamber. Either the total charge produced or the total charge produced per unit time is measured. If the gas ionized is air and if the radiation consists of photons, it is conventional to speak of exposure. This quantity, exposure, is defined as the total positive or negative charge liberated by photons in a unit mass of air. If the total charge produced is measured, the quantity found is exposure. If the charge per unit time is measured, the quantity found is the exposure rate. The concept of exposure is more fully described in Chapter 5.

Described next are some typical ion-chamber monitors, all of which are manufactured by the Victoreen Instrument Company. Similar instruments are available from other manufacturers. For precise measurements the readings obtained must be corrected for temperature and pressure.

Condenser r-Meter

The condenser r-meter is probably the most reliable and accurate instrument for measuring cumulative photon exposures. Its energy-dependence characteristics are excellent. In addition, its precision is so good that it is often used as a secondary standard for calibrating exposure values. As illustrated in Figure 3.1, this instrument consists

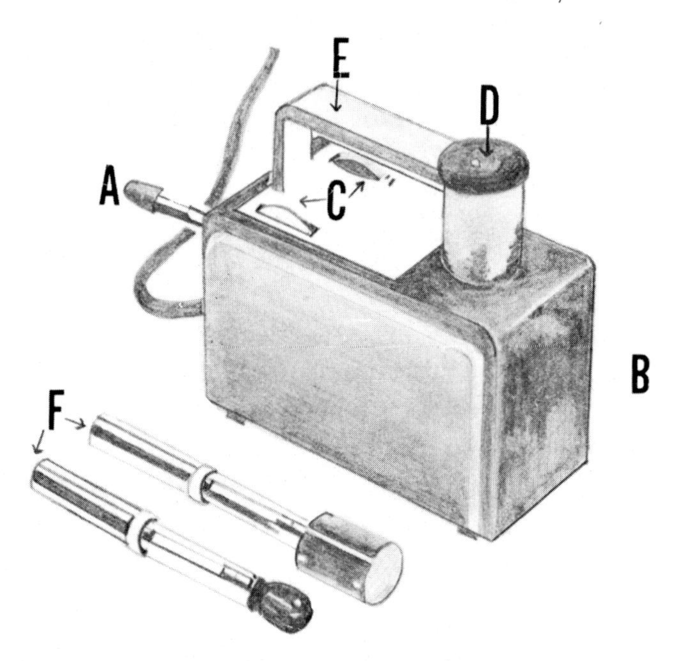

Figure 3.1: A Typical Condenser r-Meter: The ionization chamber (A) is inserted into the slot provided on the charger-reader (B). The control knobs (C) are adjusted, and the voltage is read using the microscope eyepiece (D). The device has a handle (E) for easy carrying and several different ionization chambers (F) for different energy regions and different counting rates.

of (1) a device known as a charger-reader and (2) several detachable ionization chambers.

The charger-reader has a slot into which the ion chamber is inserted. The user charges the chamber until the reading on the meter viewed through the microscope eyepiece is zero. This reading indicates that the chamber is fully charged. The chamber is then exposed to x- or gamma-ray photons and reinserted in the slot. The charger-reader measures the voltage, and the meter reading indicates the exposure value.

In the condenser r-meter the chamber is a simple electrometer, with the center electrode and the chamber walls receiving different charges. The chambers, which are made of air-equivalent material (usually Bakelite or nylon), are shaped like a thimble and thus are often referred to as "thimble chambers." Since it is desirable for all the ion pairs to be produced exclusively in the air filling the chamber, different size chambers with different wall thicknesses are needed for photons of different energies. At present three chambers are available for the following energy regions:

Low energy	6 to 35 keV
Medium energy	30 to 400 keV
High energy	400 to 1300 keV

Within each energy range, various chambers are available for different radiation source strengths.

An ion chamber with a suitable energy range and total-exposure measuring capability is selected and charged in the appropriate slot of the charger-reader. After the chamber is exposed to radiation, the exposure value is read from the meter using the eyepiece. These chambers are accurate within ±2 to ±10% provided they are properly used.

Fluoroscopic Survey Meter

The Victoreen Model 666 Fluoroscopic Survey Meter has been chosen by the Bureau of Radiological Health as the standard monitor for compliance with the Nationwide Evaluation of X-Ray Trends (NEXT) and x-ray compliance programs. It is designed to check the requirements set forth in National Bureau of Standards (NBS) Handbook 76 for monitoring fluoroscopic, dental, and other x-ray installations. Although this instrument detects x- and gamma-ray photons only, an extremely desirable combination of features and instrument capability enhance its use as a general survey and dosimetry monitor.

This instrument can be used as either an exposure (integrating) meter or an exposure rate meter. It has two probes—a background and a diagnostic probe. Each is capable of near (2 feet) or remote (20 feet) operation, and each has a broad energy response range—from 20 keV to 1.2 MeV with an accuracy of ±10% for the background probe and ±20% for the diagnostic probe. The meter has little zero drift and is temperature independent over a wide range.

"Cutie Pie"

Another instrument often used for survey work is known as the "Cutie Pie" (Fig. 3.2). Although this

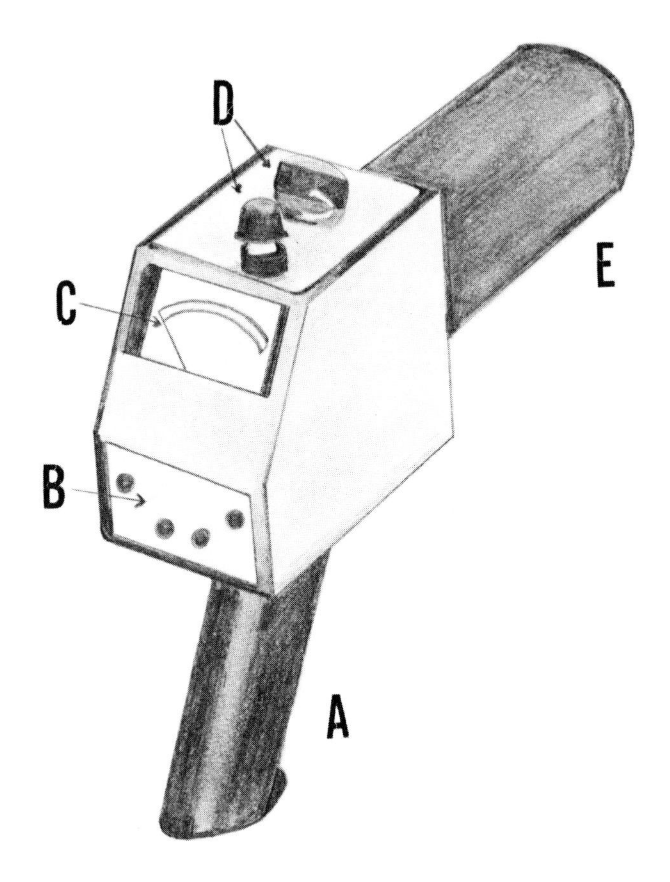

Figure 3.2: A Typical "Cutie Pie"-Type Survey Meter. This instrument has a stand (A), a multiplier selector switch (B), an easily read meter (C), and control knobs (D). Only one ionization chamber (E) is affixed directly to the front of the instrument.

name is a trademark of the Victoreen Instrument Company, as often happens, it is commonly applied to any ionization chamber with similar characteristics. Generally speaking, Cutie Pies are air-filled and measure exposure rates. These chambers usually detect only photons, but some have been modified to measure beta particles as well. The modification consists in making a thin "end-window," usually 2 to 3 microns thick, which allows beta particles to enter the chamber. Cutie Pies have quite adequate energy-dependence characteristics but low sensitivity. They can, however, detect relatively high exposure rates and, on the whole, are useful for monitoring radiation exposure rates from a wide variety of sources.

Other Meters

Some other ionization chambers used for special purposes deserve mention. The Samson meter has very thin windows for alpha-particle monitoring. The Juno meter has removable shields, which allow the user to discriminate between alpha and either beta or gamma radiation or both. The Radgun is constructed of steel and filled with high-pressure argon gas for use in both beta and gamma monitoring. This instrument, however, takes a relatively long time to respond to the presence of a source of radiation.

GEIGER-MÜLLER-TYPE MONITORS

Geiger-Müller tubes are extremely useful for monitoring low-level beta and gamma radiation. Because the tubes can be made in virtually any size or shape and because of their high sensitivity, they are the meters of choice for monitoring contamination and for searching for lost radiation sources. Most G-M tubes are equipped with an audible sound system, which is especially desirable because the user does not need to read the meter continuously in order to be aware of or to locate a radiation source.

G-M tubes are used to monitor for both beta

particles and photons. On the whole, these tubes are operated in pulse mode; consequently, the measuring apparatus takes the form of a count-rate meter with meter readings usually given in counts per minute (cpm). The relatively long dead time of G-M tubes makes them unsuitable for accurate counting at high counting rates.

CALIBRATION OF SURVEY MONITORS

All survey monitors are calibrated by the manufacturer at the time of production. Nevertheless, changes in the characteristics of the individual components of instruments may cause a change in instrument response. It is, therefore, essential that all survey meters be calibrated periodically to ensure proper reading. This calibration is especially important for G-M tubes because of their poor energy-dependence characteristics. It is recommended that Geiger-Müller-type survey meters be calibrated quarterly and after each battery exchange. They should, in any event, be calibrated at least half-yearly.

Geiger-Müller-type survey meters are calibrated using a fixed geometric arrangement between the radiation source and the detector. The radiation source most generally used is a known quantity of radiation of the same type and energy as the radiation to be monitored. Frequently, needle-like sources of ^{137}Cs are used for photons. The calibration technique should approximate the conditions under which the instrument is used. Frequently, Geiger counters have a selector switch that allows the user to set the meter to read a suitable maximum counting rate. It is important to calibrate the meter over the entire scale on each count-rate setting to compensate for any counting-rate dependence. The distance between the Geiger counter and the radiation source is varied in order to obtain different count rates. This effect of distance is discussed more fully in Chapter 7. A typical calibration geometry is shown in Figure 3.3.

All in all, survey instruments, though low in cost compared to the other instruments used in the

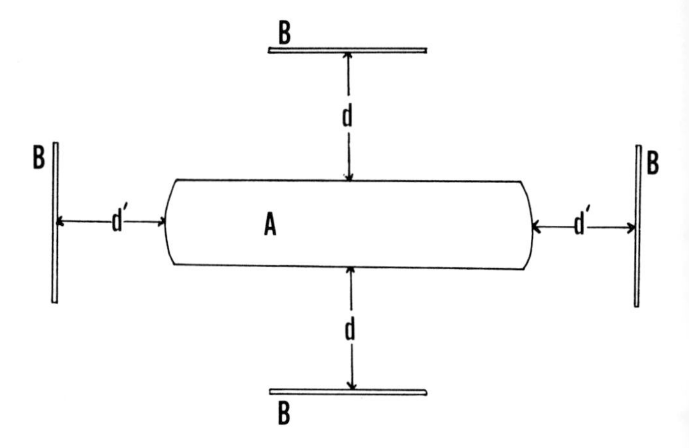

Figure 3.3: Typical Calibration Geometry from a Geiger-Müller Tube. The tube (A) is positioned symmetrically between the Standard 137 Cs needles (B).

radiologic and health field, are an important part of a good radiation safety program. It is important that no laboratory be without one. It is equally important that such monitors be used properly. The early detection of a radiation hazard can be instrumental in the prevention of unnecessary exposure to the radiation worker.

BIBLIOGRAPHY

Arena, V.: Radiation dose and radiation exposure of the human population (Chapter 9). *In* Ionizing Radiation and Life. St. Louis, The C. V. Mosby Co., 1971.

Shapiro, J.: Radiation measurement (Part IV). *In* Radiation Protection. Cambridge, MA, Harvard University Press, 1972.

Simmons, G. H., and Alexander, G. W.: Radiation protection instrumentation (Chapter XIV). *In* A Training Manual for Nuclear Medicine Technologists. Rockville, MD, U.S. Department of Health, Education and Welfare, Public Health Service, Bureau of Radiological Health, October, 1970.

chapter 4

Personnel Monitors

Determination of a person's exposure to ionizing radiation is an important function of radiation protection in general and is particularly necessary for radiation workers.

GENERAL CHARACTERISTICS OF PERSONNEL MONITORS

A personnel monitor should be reasonably accurate and reliable. It should be sensitive to the type of radiation being monitored. Furthermore, since every radiation worker should have one, personnel monitors should be cheap, portable (ideally, clipped to some article of clothing), and easy to understand (require no technical knowledge of the user). The last two are most crucial because they allow radiation workers to go about their ordinary tasks without being conscious of the personnel monitor. Hence radiation workers' ordinary exposure can be evaluated in their working environment.

Three different types of monitors are commonly used for this purpose: film badges, thermoluminescent dosimeters, and pocket dosimeters.

FILM BADGES

Undoubtedly the most popular type of personnel monitoring device is the film badge (Fig. 4.1). The film itself consists of a photographic emulsion mounted in plastic. This plastic-mounted film is wrapped in thin, light-tight paper, sandwich fashion

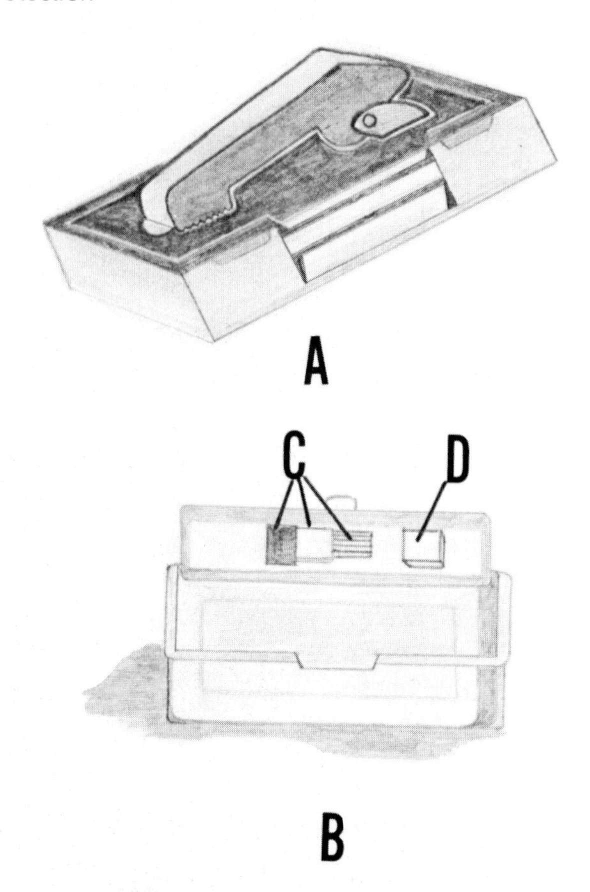

Figure 4.1: The Film Badge: (A) shows the assembled film packet and plastic case; (B) shows a cut-away view of the plastic case exposing metallic filters (C) and hole (D) for the passage of beta particles.

and placed in a plastic holder. The holder clips onto the wearer's clothing, enabling the film badge to give a measure of total, or whole-body, exposure. The plastic case usually contains a cutaway portion to allow the entrance of beta particles. It also contains three small metallic filters—usually copper, cadmium, and aluminum—placed in different portions of the case to help distinguish among higher energy photons. Each of the metals attenuates photons of different energy values. In summary, this packaging has been devised so that the film badge can give a measure of exposure of the wearer and can also help distinguish the type of radiation to which he is exposed. The outside of the film wrapper has the name, date of issue, and identification number of the wearer imprinted on it.

Although the film badge is sensitive, it does not record very low levels of exposure. However, some film badges are made with two pieces of film instead of one, one piece to detect very low levels of radiation and the other to detect even very high levels of radiation. In general, such an elaborate badge is not necessary because the lower levels of radiation not recorded on the film are insignificant, and very high levels of exposure are better monitored in other ways. As an example, a radiographer whose main work involves exposure to ionizing radiation at therapeutic levels should wear an ion-chamber pocket dosimeter as well as a film badge.

Advantages and Disadvantages

Film badges are a popular personnel monitoring device because they provide a permanent record of each individual's accumulated exposure. They are also cheap, costing between 50 cents and $1.50 apiece, and require no technical knowledge of the user. Generally speaking, employers who use film badges for their personnel monitoring contract with a separate concern to supply film badges and to collect and evaluate used ones. The contractor then gives film-badge readings to the employer, who in turn passes the information on to the radiation workers. This multistep procedure takes time, so film-badge results arrive 1 month or more after the period during which the badge is worn. Whether the film is developed in-house or by a supplier, its advantage is the permanent record thus provided. If necessary, film can be reread. This rereading capability offers a distinct advantage because, if a mistake is made, particularly if the reading is too high, a person may have to leave his job. (The limitations on personal exposure are discussed in Chapter 6.) The film badge is the only personnel monitoring device that has this advantage. It should be mentioned, however, that film is not accurate for any exact measurement purpose. Film can give only an indication of radiation level. It also has low reproducibility.

The film badge operates in the following way. When radiation is absorbed in the film emulsion, some of the silver halide grains that compose it are altered. These altered grains then respond differently to the reducing agents, known as developers; i.e., those grains affected by radiation are reduced to metallic silver at a faster rate than grains that were not so affected. This developable state produced in the emulsion by the action of radiation is called the latent image. The optical density of developed film, i.e., its degree of darkening, is proportional to the exposure of the film (Fig. 4.2). The relationship between exposure and density is determined by comparison with films exposed to known amounts of radiation of the same energy, since optical density produced by a given exposure of radiation is strongly dependent upon the energy of that radiation. It should be noted that photographic emulsions

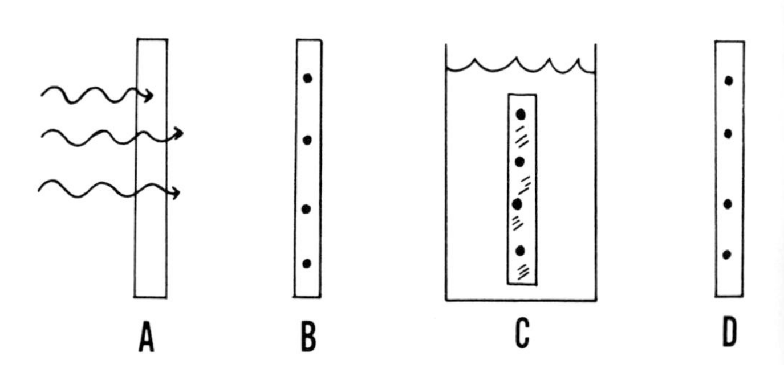

Figure 4.2: Radiation and Film: A shows the radiation passing through the emulsion activating some of the grains and thus forming the latent image B. The development stage C reduces the emulsion and produces, in D, visible grains. These last contain the image or the record of passage of the ionizing particles. (Courtesy Donald J. Pizzarello.)

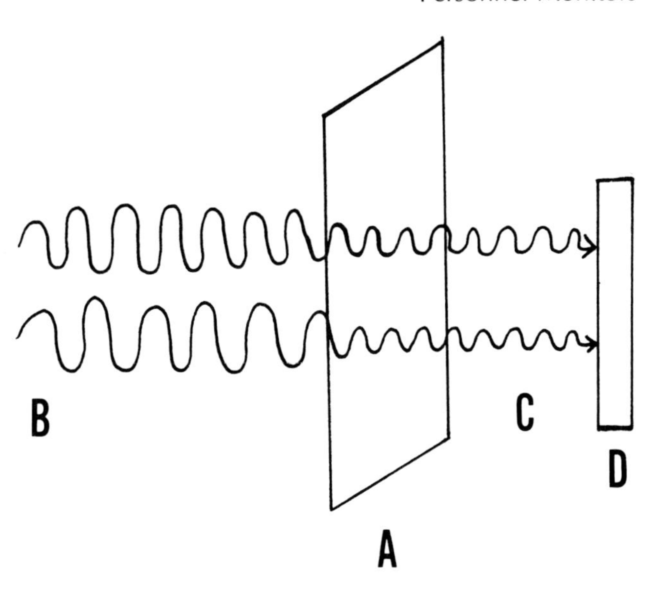

Figure 4.3: Metal filters (A), generally by means of Compton interactions, attenuate the original photons (B) and create photons (C) of lower energy. The film (D) is more sensitive to these lower energy photons.

are much more sensitive to low-energy radiation than to high. It is, therefore, useful to include metallic filters because these attenuate higher energy photons in varying degrees, thus lowering their energy to a value more suitable for detection by the film. By looking at the resulting density variation of the film, the reader is able to estimate the energy of radiation to which the film was exposed (Fig. 4.3).

Precautions

Because the film badge is essentially a photographic device, two basic precautions apply:

1. Heat affects film; hence the badge should not be exposed to sunlight or stored in a warm place such as an automobile (because of the greenhouse effect).

2. The latent image begins to fade after a time, so a piece of film should not be used for more than 1

or 2 months before developing. General practice dictates that film badges be replaced biweekly or monthly. For the radiologic and health sciences where radiation levels are low, a monthly change of film badge is sufficient. Cost, as well as insensitivity of film to very low levels of radiation, prohibits changing of film badges at more frequent intervals.

It is common in many laboratories and clinics to have one extra film badge placed in some generally unexposed portion of the room or department. This badge, viewed as a control, is then developed with those of the employees. It serves to separate exposure due to background levels of radiation from exposures an individual radiation worker may acquire as a result of his work habits. In this way high background levels can be detected and eliminated, and careless radiation workers can be admonished.

Types

Radiation workers who regularly use radionuclides usually wear a ring badge on one of their fingers in addition to a badge clipped to their clothing. This is because their hands are often in near contact with photon-emitting substances as they perform tasks such as milking the generator, preparing necessary radiopharmaceuticals and doses, and injecting patients. Ring badges monitor the exposure of hands specifically rather than the whole body. Ring badges can, of course, be made of film. Other special-purpose badges, such as wrist badges, also exist for monitoring particular areas of the body. An alternative to film for both whole-body monitoring and special-purpose monitoring is a recent invention known as the thermoluminescent dosimeter.

THERMOLUMINESCENT DOSIMETERS (TLD's)

These personnel monitors can be used like film badges. They are common for whole-body monitoring as well as for special types of monitoring, such as that described for hands.

Substances that possess the property of thermoluminescence are nonmetallic crystalline solids, usually in powdered form. A crystal is an aggregate of atoms of one or more elements put together in a distinctive way. When carbon exists in crystalline form, it is known as diamond. When it exists in noncrystalline form, it is called graphite and is used for lead pencils. Ordinary table salt is a crystal, but its crystalline structure does not have the property of thermoluminescence.

Electrons in a crystal exist in distinct energy levels, called bands, just as electrons in an atom exist in distinct energy levels, called orbits. When electrons in a crystal absorb energy, they move to a higher energy band. In a thermoluminescent crystal, these excited electrons get trapped in a higher energy state until the crystal is heated to a specific (usually high) temperature. At that temperature, the electrons return to their normal or ground state, radiating their extra energy in the form of visible light photons, hence the name, thermal (heat) luminescent (light-giving). Lithium fluoride (LiF) is a crystal commonly used for its thermoluminescent properties.

Personnel monitors contain a thermoluminescent powder, or other unique solid-state form such as a ribbon, which is molded into a shape appropriate for its function. When a thermoluminescent substance is exposed to ionizing radiation, electrons in the crystalline structure of the material are excited to higher energy states. A certain number of these excited electrons get trapped in what are known as sensitivity centers. When the crystals are heated, the electrons return to the ground state, and the excitation energy appears in the form of visible light. The amount of light obtained is proportional to the energy absorbed by the crystal. If the crystal is then annealed properly, in other words, slowly cooled allowing it to relieve stress in its lattice as the temperature is brought down, the crystal structure is not damaged, and the powder, or whatever, is ready for use again.

So, one advantage of thermoluminescent dosimeters is that they can be reused. It is relatively easy to determine an exposure value from such a device because all that is required is an oven and a light meter. Since the crystalline structure and energy levels of the substance used are well known, a direct measurement of energy absorbed is obtained. Also thermoluminescent dosimeters are not as sensitive to moderate heat as is film, nor do they suffer from fading of information. Furthermore, when compared to film, they have an increased sensitivity to a wide photon energy range. TLD's can be used for several weeks at a time without appreciable loss of stored energy. Most important, they require no technical knowledge for use.

Disadvantages of TLD's include higher cost than that for a film badge and, more significantly, a nonpermanent record of exposure. Once the TLD has been heated and annealed, the information is gone. Recently, some researchers have attempted to eliminate this reproducibility problem.

Thermoluminescent dosimeters are excellent monitors and are enjoying a well-deserved popularity.

Other chemicals, such as radioluminescent substances, are also used for monitoring. However, they are not commonly used for monitoring in the radiologic and health fields so they will not be discussed.

ION-CHAMBER PERSONNEL MONITORS

In addition to the monitors just discussed, one more type has been designed so that exposure levels can be read at any time, either by the user or by some other designated person. These simple ion-chamber monitors are shaped like a large fountain pen and attached to the clothing (Fig. 4.4). As with other ionization chambers, these monitors must be calibrated for energy range of the radiation to be monitored as well as for permissible amount of charge leakage per week for the chamber to remain in calibration. If the barrel of the chamber is made of

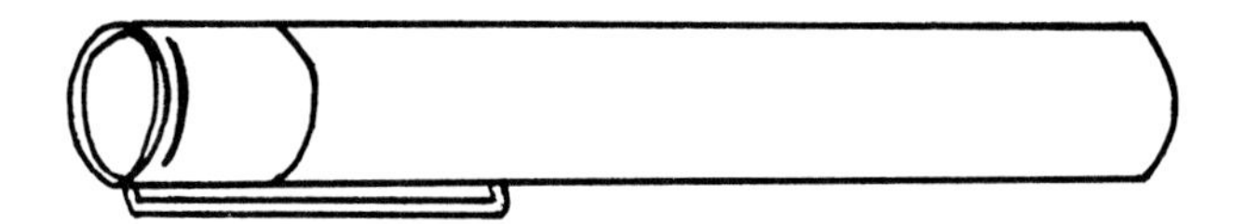

Figure 4.4: Typical Ionization Chamber Personnel Monitor.

aluminum, another correction factor may also have to be employed.

Two kinds of ion-chamber monitors are available. One is known as a self-reading pocket monitor because the person using it can take a reading at any time. The other is a condenser-type pocket chamber. The latter requires a separate device for both charging and obtaining results. A brief description of each type is given next.

Self-Reading Monitors

This monitor is an ionization chamber containing two central electrodes, one of which is fixed. The other electrode is a quartz fiber loop that is free to move with respect to its mounting. Placing like charges on the electrodes results in a repulsive force between the two, which forces the loop outward from the mount. The ionization produced in the chamber by external radiation, particularly photons, reduces the charge and allows the fiber to move toward its normal position. This action is similar to that of an electroscope, which is commonly used for measuring charge (see Glossary).

The self-reading monitor is cylindrical in shape. One end is made of glass to allow light to enter; a transparent scale forms the other end. The instrument is read by simply holding it up to light. The quartz fiber casts a shadow on the scale, which is calibrated in exposure units. Hence the user can determine exposure immediately.

This kind of ion chamber is particularly useful for monitoring personnel such as doctors and nurses who are caring for hospitalized patients receiving therapeutic levels of radiation. These therapeutic treatments involve either radioactive implants or large doses of radionuclides such as ^{131}I. In this case, each person entering the patient's room is required to wear a pocket chamber while in the room. A log is placed outside the patient's room. Each person logs the chamber's reading before entering the room, then again when leaving. Each person also logs his name, the date, and the amount of time spent in the patient's room.

Condenser-Type Pocket Chambers

The condenser-type pocket chamber has a central wire and a cylindrical electrode insulated from a Bakelite wall (Bakelite is used because it is light, hard, effective as an insulator, and heat resistant). A charge is placed on the center electrode by means of an external charging unit. Ions formed in the chamber reduce the charge by an amount proportional to the radiation exposure. The condenser-type pocket chamber differs from the self-reading kind mainly in that the functions performed by the quartz fiber and scale mechanism are in an external unit. Consequently, the chamber must be read with a separate charger-reader, similar to that described in Chapter 3.

The advantage of condenser-type pocket chambers over self-reading ones is that they are lower in price. The condenser type is most often used for monitoring radiation oncology personnel, such as technicians and physicians, because of their high probability of being exposed to substantial amounts of radiation. Should the necessity arise, the amount of exposure incurred could be determined immediately. Both kinds of ion-chamber devices must be recharged daily since significant leakage of charge may occur over long periods of time. Both kinds are read immediately after use. In addition, ion-chamber monitors tend to be fragile rather than rugged.

The ion-chamber type of personnel monitor is more costly than either the thermoluminescent dosimeter or the film badge, with the condenser type of ion chamber being less expensive than the self-reading kind. However, self-reading ion-chamber personnel monitors can be read immediately. It does take a certain amount of skill to do the reading, but the user can easily gain this capability. The condenser type does not require any skill to use. Because they should be read daily, ion-chamber personnel monitors are not necessary for monitoring persons who may be exposed only to very low levels of radiation. As with thermoluminescent dosimeters, ion chambers leave no permanent record of the user's exposure. Once readings are taken and values recorded (or possibly not recorded), double-checking is not possible.

In summary then, all personnel who may be exposed to even very low levels of radiation need to be monitored. This monitoring can be accomplished in a number of ways. The particular method chosen depends on the type and level of radiation to which the user is most frequently exposed as well as the cost and dependability of the monitoring method.

BIBLIOGRAPHY

Arena, V.: Radiation dose and radiation exposure of the human population (Chapter 9). *In* Ionizing Radiation and Life. St. Louis, The C. V. Mosby Co., 1971.

Shapiro, J.: Radiation measurements (Part IV). *In* Radiation Protection. Cambridge, MA, Harvard University Press, 1972.

Simmons, G. H., and Alexander, G. W.: Radiation protection instrumentation (Chapter XIV). *In* A Training Manual for Nuclear Medicine Technologists. Rockville, MD, U.S. Dept. of Health, Education and Welfare, Public Health Service, Bureau of Radiological Health, October 1970.

chapter 5

The Units of Radiation Protection

When living cells are exposed to ionizing radiation, they may absorb some or all of the energy carried by the ionizing radiation. The energy transferred from ionizing radiation to living cells is what damages them. The amount of radiation to which living cells are exposed is referred to as exposure, and the amount of energy actually absorbed from radiation by living cells is known as dose. Except in the case of photons, exposure and dose are for all practical purposes the same. However, for ionizing radiation consisting mainly of photons, it is necessary to study in detail the distinction between exposure and dose and also to see how they are related. In brief, exposure is a property of photons, namely their ability to ionize air, and absorbed dose describes the energy taken from any ionizing radiation. It is necessary also to understand how the unit of dose is defined and how it is related to biologic damage in humans.

THE UNIT OF EXPOSURE

For low-energy photons of the type encountered in the radiologic and health sciences, a special unit of exposure has been defined. This unit is based on the ionization of air and is determined using a special detector known as a standard ionization chamber. This chamber is analogous to the standard

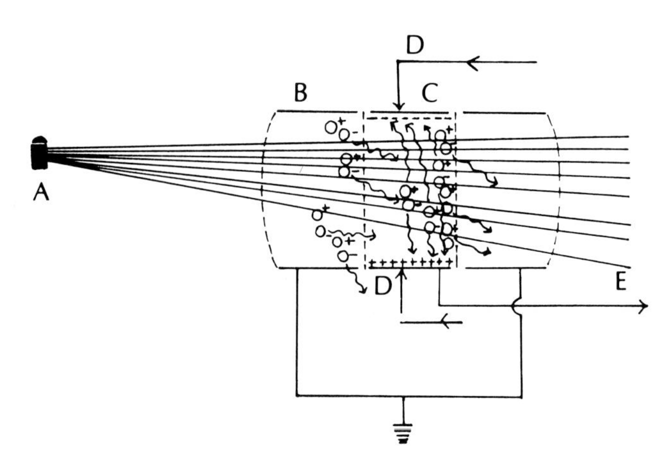

Figure 5.1: Outline of a Standard Ion Chamber. The photons are emitted by the source (A) and enter the outer cell (B), which is grounded. The inner cell (C) is surrounded on both sides by air-filled grounded cells. Ions are collected on the electrodes (D), which are connected (E) to a charge sensitive measuring device. (Adapted from Johns, H.E., and Cunningham, J.R.: The Physics of Radiology, 3rd ed. Springfield, IL, Charles C Thomas, Publisher, 1974.)

meter stick,* a bar of platinum-iridium alloy kept at the International Bureau of Weights and Measures at Sèvres, near Paris. This bar is maintained at carefully controlled temperature and pressure conditions to ensure that its length does not change.

During the French Revolution the need for international standards was realized. The standards then developed for length and mass, kept in the museum, were placed there during the reign of the Emperor Napoleon. The standard ionization chamber (Fig. 5.1) is a similar reference, from which all other ion chambers are calibrated.

When a beam of photons passes through matter, not all the photons interact. The unit of exposure is based upon the amount of charge released by

*Note that today the standard for length is defined in terms of one wavelength of krypton-86 (^{86}Kr) instead of the standard meter stick.

photons as they pass through a specified mass of air. In general, 1 unit of exposure is designated as 1 coulomb (C); i.e., 1 unit of positive or negative charge, released in a kilogram of air:

$$1 \text{ exposure unit} = 1 \text{ C kg}^{-1} \text{ (air)} \qquad (5.1)$$

This equation reflects the way the unit of exposure is defined in the International System (SI) of units.†

In the old system of units, 1 exposure unit was defined somewhat differently and was known as 1 roentgen (see Appendix II). As can be seen from Figure 5.1, the standard ion chamber is composed of a unit cell of air with electrodes placed on two sides (top and bottom in diagram). Surrounding the unit cell are similar air-filled cells, but without electrodes in them.

Consider a beam of photons moving from left to right, as shown in Figure 5.1. Photons pass through the first cell on the left, ionizing some air molecules along their path and thus producing electrons. As long as these electrons do not enter the central cell, they cannot reach the electrode. However, some electrons formed outside the central cell do enter it and do reach the electrodes. These electrons give a false exposure value (they add to the number of coulombs collected on the central electrode, which ideally collects only electrons produced in the volume of the central cell) unless there is some way to compensate for them. At the same time, some of the electrons produced by ionization in the central cell pass into the cell to the right before they can be collected on the electrode. It would be convenient if the number of electrons entering the central cell from the left were equal to the number of electrons leaving to the right. When such a situation exists, it

†SI units will be used throughout this text; consequently, 1 exposure unit will simply be referred to as 1 coulomb per kilogram of air. This international standard of units was adopted by the International Commission on Radiation Units and Measurements (ICRU) in order to bring research work and applications in the radiologic and health sciences into conformity with the units being used in other scientific fields.

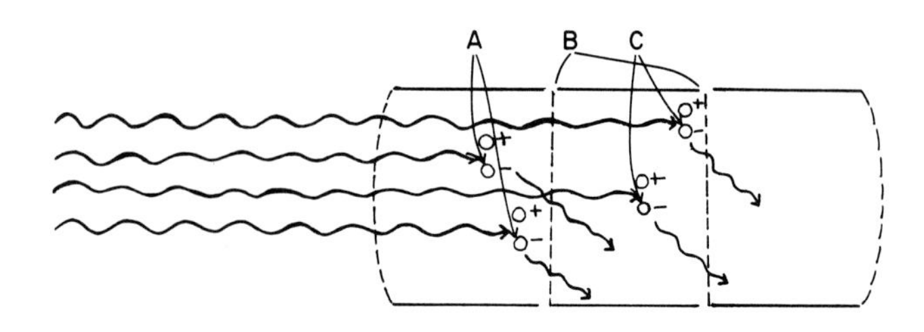

Figure 5.2: Electron Equilibrium. The electrons (A), although produced outside the standard cell (B), enter it. The electrons (C), although produced in the standard cell, leave it. For electron equilibrium to hold, the number of electrons (A) must be equal to the number of electrons (C). (Adapted from Johns, H. E., and Cunningham, J. R.: The Physics of Radiology, 3rd ed. Springfield, IL, Charles C Thomas, Publisher, 1974.)

is known as electron equilibrium (Fig. 5.2). Unfortunately, the determination of exposure values using the standard ion chamber is valid only when electron equilibrium can be established. Since the density of air is small, higher energy photons do not readily interact with it. In fact, it is only possible to define exposure values for photon energies up to about 3 MeV. Generally speaking, exposure units are an accurate measure only for photon energies between 1 keV and 1000 keV (1 MeV).

Ion chambers, which are used to determine exposure values from radition therapy machines, are usually sent to a special center, where they are calibrated using a standard ionization chamber. Several such centers exist in the United States. Among them are the Sloan Kettering Institute in New York City, the National Bureau of Standards in Washington, D.C., and the Victoreen Company Center near Cleveland, Ohio.

Remember that the exposure unit is defined only for photons. This restriction limits the usefulness of the exposure unit considerably. The following units are defined for all kinds of ionizing radiation.

THE UNIT OF ABSORBED DOSE

The pathway of ionizing radiation through matter is marked by a transfer of energy from radiation to the material through which it passes. Such transfer of energy is typical of all kinds of ionizing radiation and not restricted just to photons. The amount of energy transferred is known as the absorbed energy, or the absorbed dose. The unit of absorbed energy, or dose, is called a gray (Gy), after a physicist of that name who was instrumental in establishing experimental techniques to measure absorbed energy.

A gray is defined as 1 joule (J) of energy absorbed from any ionizing radiation in 1 kilogram (kg) of any material. In symbolic form,

$$1\ \text{Gy} = 1\ \text{J kg}^{-1} \tag{5.2}$$

The older unit of absorbed dose, known as the rad, is discussed in Appendix II. A rad and a gray are very simply related:

$$1\ \text{rad} = 10^{-2}\text{Gy} \tag{5.3}$$

Therefore, any dose values expressed in rads can be expressed in grays simply by dividing by 100. Many of the tables of absorbed dose are expressed in terms of rads. Since survey meters and personnel monitors measure exposure, it is important to see the relationship between the quantities of exposure and of absorbed dose. This relationship, as mentioned previously, applies only to photons. The equivalence between exposure and dose is found in the following manner. Whenever it is necessary to change units, e.g., from energy expressed in units of electron volts to energy expressed in units of joules, one should keep in mind that, whenever something is multiplied by one, nothing is changed. To illustrate this point.

$$1\ \text{eV} = 1.6 \cdot 10^{-19}\text{J} \tag{5.4}$$

Divide both sides of equation 5.4 by 1 eV. Then

$$\frac{1\ \text{eV}}{1\ \text{eV}} = 1 = \frac{1.6 \cdot 10^{-19}\text{J}}{1\ \text{eV}} \qquad (5.5)$$

Consequently, $1.6 \cdot 10^{-19}\text{J eV}^{-1}$ is equivalent to one; therefore, it can be multiplied by any equation.

When one air molecule is ionized, an electron is produced which carries a negative charge of $1.6 \cdot 10^{-19}$ coulombs. The residual ion carries the same charge, except that it is positive. Accordingly,

$$1\ \text{ion pr} = 1.6 \cdot 10^{-19}\text{C} \qquad (5.6)$$

At the same time, it takes 34 eV of energy to ionize one molecule of air.

Essentially then, the problem is to find out how many joules of energy must be absorbed to produce 1 coulomb of charge.

$$1\ \text{exp unit} = \frac{1\text{C}}{\text{kg}} \cdot \frac{1\ \text{ion pr}}{1.6 \cdot 10^{-19}\text{C}} \cdot \frac{34\text{eV}}{\text{ion pr}} \cdot \frac{1.6 \cdot 10^{-19}\text{J}}{\text{eV}} \cdot \frac{1\text{Gy} \cdot \text{kg}}{\text{J}} = 34\ \text{Gy} \qquad (5.7)$$

In brief, the important point is:

$$1\ \text{exp unit} = 1\ \text{C kg}^{-1} = 34\ \text{Gy (in air)} \qquad (5.8)$$

The unit of absorbed dose just defined applies to any material. Although all ionizing radiation can produce similar biologic effects, the absorbed dose necessary to produce a particular effect may vary from one kind of radiation to another and from one type of biologic material to another.

BIOLOGIC EFFECTS

The ratio of the absorbed dose of photons of a specified energy to the absorbed dose of any other ionizing radiation required to produce the same biologic effect is called the Relative Biological Effectiveness (RBE). For example, suppose that an absorbed dose of 0.2 Gy, or 20 rads, from slow neutrons produces the same biologic damage as 1.0 Gy, or 100 rads, from photons of a specific energy. Then the RBE for slow neutrons in this example is:

$$\text{RBE} = \frac{1\ \text{Gy}}{0.2\ \text{Gy}} = 5 \tag{5.9}$$

Apparently then, slow neutrons are five times as damaging as photons.

The RBE of any particular kind of ionizing radiation is a function not only of the energy of the radiation but also of the type and degree of biologic damage and the nature of the tissue or organism under consideration. As a consequence, it is more practical for radiation protection work to use a quantity known as the quality factor (Q).

This quality factor is defined as an average RBE factor based on the macroscopic effects of radiation on the human organism. The Q or quality factor is used in setting radiation protection standards, and the RBE is generally reserved for radiobiologic work where more precise values are needed. Table 5.1 gives a list of more commonly encountered ionizing radiations and their associated quality factors.

Table 5.1

Quality Factors (Q) for Some Ionizing Radiations

Ionizing Radiation	Q
Photons	1
Beta particles > 0.03 MeV	1
Beta particles < 0.03 MeV	1.7
Protons	10
Alpha particles	10
Fast neutrons	10
Thermal neutrons	3
Heavy ions	20

Reproduced with permission of the U.S. Department of Health, Education and Welfare, Public Health Service, Food and Drug Administration, Bureau of Radiological Health, from the Radiological Health Handbook, rev. ed., 1970.

EFFECTS IN MAN

Finally, there is a special unit which applies absorbed doses specifically to man. It is known as the sievert,* which is defined as absorbed dose in grays multiplied by RBE.

$$\text{Absorbed dose in sieverts} = \text{Absorbed dose in grays} \cdot \text{RBE} \quad (5.10)$$

Again, radiation protection work uses a quantity called the dose equivalent, which is defined in terms of the quality factor.

$$\text{Dose equivalent} = \text{Absorbed dose in grays} \cdot \text{quality factor} \cdot \text{other modifying factors} \quad (5.11)$$

Symbolically,

$$H = D \cdot Q \cdot N$$

where H is dose equivalent, D is absorbed dose, Q is quality factor, and N is other modifying factors. In the case of an external radiation source, N is defined as one.

Since the Q for photons is one, the absorbed dose and the dose equivalent are equal provided N is also one. In the radiologic and health sciences, photons and high-energy beta particles are the most frequent, and often only, types of ionizing radiation encountered. As a result, for most practical purposes, dose equivalent and absorbed dose can be treated as the same quantity.

*The sievert (Sv) is named for a Swedish physicist of that name who has done much work in this field. The sievert has not yet been officially adopted by the International Bureau of Weights & Measures in Paris (BIPM) which sets the SI units. However, it is unlikely that this body will consider the sievert since it is a very specialized unit. The ICRU, which is charged with defining the units used in radiation applications, has adopted the sievert, and it is in use by the International Commission on Radiological Protection (ICRP) and the National Council on Radiation Protection and Measurements (NCRP).

In the old system of measurement, the special unit that applies the absorbed dose specifically to man is known as the rem, a mnemonic for Roentgen Equivalent Man. The rem is defined as absorbed dose in rads times RBE:

$$\text{rem} = \text{rads} \cdot \text{RBE} \tag{5.12}$$

In the old system, the dose equivalent H was also defined:

$$\text{H (rems)} = \text{D (rads)} \cdot \text{Q} \cdot \text{N} \tag{5.13}$$

BIBLIOGRAPHY

Arena, V.: Radiation dose and radiation exposure of the human population (Chapter 9). *In* Ionizing Radiation and Life. St. Louis, The C. V. Mosby Co., 1971.

Johns, H. E., and Cunningham, J. R.: The measurement of radiation (Chapter VII). *In* The Physics of Radiology. 3rd ed. Springfield, IL, Charles C Thomas, Publisher, 1973.

Lidin, K.: Communication. Med. Phys. 3:52, 1976.

Shapiro, J.: Principles of radiation protection (Part II). *In* Radiation Protection. Cambridge, MA, Harvard University Press, 1972.

Simmons, G. H., and Alexander, G. W.: Units of radiation exposure and dose (Chapter XIII). *In* A Training Manual for Nuclear Medicine Technologists. Rockville, MD, U.S. Department of Health, Education and Welfare, Public Health Service, Bureau of Radiological Health, October, 1970.

chapter 6

MAXIMUM PERMISSIBLE DOSE

When ionizing radiation was discovered, it was not known whether it might be dangerous. Over the years, much evidence has been accumulated to document that ionizing radiation is not only dangerous but also lethal in some situations. The lower limit on the radiation dose that will cause death in a very short time is the subject of a great deal of research. What concerns scientists, in particular, radiobiologists, even more is whether very low levels of radiation dose extended over a relatively long time cause adverse reactions in humans.

Several years ago, the National Academy of Sciences commissioned a study group to seek an answer to this question. The results of that study, published in 1972, are detailed in the Biological Effects of Ionizing Radiation (BEIR) report. The BEIR Committee studied in particular the fate of the early x-ray workers, the radium-dial painters (p. 69), and the atomic bomb victims of Hiroshima and Nagasaki. In their initial 1972 report the BEIR Committee found a linear relationship between radiation effects and absorbed dose (see Fig. 1.1). Curve A shows the initial report results; curve B shows the later trend, which some researchers believe to be correct. After further study, some members of the BEIR Committee concluded that the data showed no indication of any harmful effects from very low levels of absorbed doses of ionizing radiation. Curve C shows the opposite effect; i.e., low levels of radiation may be proportionately more harmful than higher levels. Which curve is actually correct is a question that will not be resolved in the near future.

Since radiation workers in the radiologic and health sciences can be routinely exposed to very low levels of radiation, for them this question is crucial. The quantitative question of what is an acceptable (safe) level of radiation exposure and, consequently, radiation dose has been attempted by a number of different commissions and committees.

REGULATORY AGENCIES

The standards for maximum exposure have been suggested by several different agencies. One, already mentioned in reference to the BEIR report, is the National Academy of Sciences; others are the International Commission on Radiological Protection (ICRP), the National Council on Radiation Protection and Measurements (NCRP), and the International Commission on Radiation Units and Measurements (ICRU). These agencies have no law-making or enforcing power; they simply make recommendations. However, based on their recommendations, limits can be set by an act of Congress or other law-making body.

In the United States, several agencies have been charged with enforcing the standards that are set. On a national level the Nuclear Regulatory Commission (NRC), formerly the Atomic Energy Commission (AEC), is in charge of regulating safety in all aspects that pertain to reactor products. Thus, the NRC would be concerned with safety in transport, possession, and use as well as worker safety. For other sources of ionizing radiation, the states themselves enforce the regulations through their health codes. In some cases, as in New York City, a city enforces the regulations under its own health code. Radiation workers are also governed by the Occupational Health and Safety Act (OHSA). The intent of OHSA is to protect the safety and health of all workers; radiologic and health workers are no exception.

In some cases the NRC has entered into an agreement with a state, known as an "agreement state," in which the NRC relinquishes its governing role with respect to reactor products to that state. In these cases, the state regulations must be at least as stringent as those of the NRC. Likewise a state has sometimes entered into an agreement with one of its cities, e.g., New York and New York City, as mentioned in the preceding paragraph.

EXPOSURE LIMITS

Limits of exposure have been set for occupationally exposed workers, nonoccupationally exposed individuals, and the population as a whole.

The amount of exposure given to an individual in the course of diagnostic or therapeutic procedures is regulated by the licensing process for facilities and physicians, and through accepted medical practice. This exposure is not included in an individual's maximum permissible dose (MPD) because the medical benefit derived from this exposure outweighs the physical risks associated with it. The MPD is stated in terms of sieverts, here defined as the dose in grays times the quality factor. To obtain the MPD in rems, simply multiply each stated limit by 100.

The average limit set for the entire population is 17 mSv per year or less. The population limit is based on the genetic risk to both an individual and the population. Because this genetic consideration is very important, it has been studied extensively. Mainly, it is the province of radiobiology to assess risks and benefits to the population as a whole from ionizing radiation. (The text by Pizzarello and Witcofski concerns this aspect of radiation.) The current risk estimates state that 0.5 Gy (50 rads) equals the genetic doubling dose, i.e., doubles the risk of genetically different offspring being produced. Remember that a certain number of mutants are born in the normal course of events. Exposure to ionizing radiation increases the frequency with which such mutants are born.

The average limit set for whole-body exposure of an occupationally exposed individual is 50 mSv per year. The MPD for different parts of the body and for the critical organs of a radiation worker are summarized in Table 6.1. A pregnant radiation worker should note that the dose limit for her fetus is 10 times lower than her own and should take proper precautions.

The total lifetime dose of a radiation worker may not exceed 50(N−18)mSv where N is the worker's age. Thus, a radiation worker must be at least 18 years old. Persons under 18 who are studying to be radiation workers must follow the MPD limit set for nonoccupationally exposed individuals; this limit is 10 times less than that for radiation workers.

In addition, the radiation worker may not accumulate in one quarter year (3 months or 13 weeks) any more than 30 mSv. In other words, if in any 3-month period a worker acquires a dose of 30 mSv, he can acquire only 20 additional mSv in the total calendar year period, i.e., the next 9 months. Since an employer is bound by law to obtain a new employee's radiation exposure record (which extends back 5 years and always includes the total lifetime dose), neither this regulation nor any other can be circumvented by a change of employer. Employees working for two different employers si-

Table 6.1

MPD for Occupationally Exposed Personnel

Occupational Exposure Limits on:	*Yearly MPD Limit in mSv*	*(rems)*
Whole body, lens of eye, red bone marrow, gonads	50	(5)
Hands and feet	750	(75)
Forearms and ankles	300	(30)
Any other specific organ not mentioned above (including skin)	150	(15)
Fetus in gestation period	5	(0.5)

Values taken from NCRP Report No. 39, 1971.

multaneously should make each employer aware of the records of the other. For his own sake a radiation worker should not try to cheat the system.

The MPD for nonoccupationally exposed individuals is 5 mSv to the whole body. Note that this figure is a factor of 10 less than that for the occupationally exposed individual. Since the radiation worker is deriving specific benefits from his exposure, namely, his livelihood, his risk should be higher.

THE USE OF MPD

The major use of the MPD limits is to derive working standards. The first standard applies to radiation facilities themselves and regulates the amount of radiation that may be present in areas where occupationally exposed personnel work and where nonoccupationally exposed people are present or work. (An example of the latter is a secretary's office or a waiting area.) By MPD standards, a radiation worker should not be exposed to more than 25 μSv per hour of radiation or to more than 4 mSv per month. Therefore, ambient radiation levels from x-ray machines or from radionuclides must be kept below this level.

The MPD also helps set the maximum permissible body burden (MPBD) from chronic ingestion. Remember the radium-dial painters: many, actually most of them, contracted leukemia as well as lung and bone cancer because they used to put a nice point on their paintbrush by placing it in their mouths. Nowadays, the dials and hands of watches and clocks are made luminescent (i.e., made to glow in the dark) by the use of materials such as tritium.

In addition, the MPD allows the determination of concentrations of radiation in air and water and other aspects of the environment. These limits are taken into consideration when facilities are in the design stage, and shielding must be planned for use in and with these facilities in order to reduce exposure and, consequently, dose to an acceptable level.

Chapter 7 details the practical methods used to reduce exposure to that acceptable level.

BIBLIOGRAPHY

Arena, V.: Radiation dose and radiation exposure of the human population (Chapter 9). *In* Ionizing Radiation and Life. St. Louis, The C. V. Mosby Co., 1971.

The Effects on Populations of Exposure to Low Levels of Ionizing Radiation. Report of the Advisory Committee on the Biological Effects of Ionizing Radiation (BEIR Reports I & II). Washington, D.C., Division of Medical Sciences, National Academy of Sciences, National Research Council, 1972 and 1977.

Pizzarello, D. J., and Witcofski, R.L.: Basic Radiation Biology, 2nd ed. Philadelphia, Lea & Febiger, 1975.

Shapiro, J.: Radiation measurement (Part VI). *In* Radiation Protection. Cambridge, MA, Harvard University Press, 1972.

Simmons, G. H., and Alexander, G. W.: Units of radiation exposure and dose (Chapter XIII). *In* A Training Manual for Nuclear Medicine Technologists. Rockville, MD, U.S. Department of Health, Education and Welfare, Public Health Service, Bureau of Radiological Health, October, 1970.

chapter 7

Practical Means of Radiation Protection

As evidence began to accumulate that exposure to ionizing radiation was inherently dangerous, practical methods of protection were developed. In essence, the three effective means of protection from ionizing radiation are time, distance, and shielding.

TIME

The simplest protection from ionizing radiation is not to be where it exists. An important principle in dealing with radiation is to spend as little time as possible in the vicinity of radiation. Translated into practical terms, this principle has several implications.

As a first example, consider ordinary radiography. It is sometimes necessary to hold a patient in place; e.g., the patient may be quite young, elderly, or ill. The technician or physician can best hold the patient; however, it would be much better for someone who is not a radiation worker to do the holding. If possible, a relative of the patient should be asked to help. The person then being exposed is exposed only once, whereas the technician or physician is constantly exposed. Recently, New York State has made illegal the practice of persons occupationally exposed to radiation (e.g., technicians) holding patients during an examination. An institution is not even allowed to hire a person for that purpose or to utilize a limited number of persons regularly. Furthermore, the institution is required to monitor, and maintain for inspection, records of exposure to *any* person holding a patient.

When it is necessary to be exposed to radiation, a good rule of thumb is to develop efficient working habits and techniques. This measure applies particularly to radionuclide work and to fluoroscopy. For example, when the Mo-Tc^{99} generator is milked in a nuclear medicine laboratory, it should be done skillfully, so that the person milking is exposed for as short a time as possible. The same applies to chemical preparations containing radionuclides, and it also applies to the preparation and administration of doses.

The less time spent in actual handling of radioactive material, the better. This rule is true even when such other protective methods as distance and shielding are used. *The best exposure is no exposure.* This same principle of skillful technique applies to fluoroscopy as well; the shorter the time during which the x-ray beam is turned on, the better. Thus the importance of respecting this protocol is evident as is the advantage of practicing new protocols without using any actual radiation.

DISTANCE

The most effective means of protection from ionizing radiation is a wise use of distance. The nice thing about distance is that particulate radiation has a very short range, even in air; as for photons, the number reaching a particular point in space decreases according to an inverse square law, as they move farther and farther away from their source.

This concept of an inverse square law requires further explanation. Picture a number cf spheres of different sizes all centered on one spot, e.g., a golf ball, a tennis ball, a bowling ball, and a basketball, all having a common center and each inside the other (Fig. 7.1).

Now picture lines drawn from the center and intercepting the surfaces of all balls. Since Figure 7.1

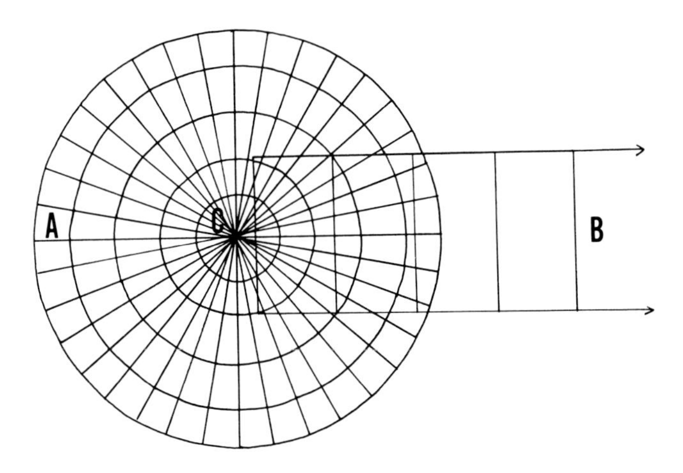

Figure 7.1: Diagram of Concept of the Inverse Square Law: The lines (A) radiating from the center (C) spread out as they go from inner circle to outer circle. If a constant length (B) is placed across the circumference (edge) of each of the circles, it is seen that fewer lines (A) are intercepted by the length (B) as it moves from the inner to the outer circles.

is drawn in two dimensions, the lines intercept the circumference or boundary of various circles. If a definite size block were then chosen and placed on the surface of each of the balls (or boundary of each of the circles), the number of lines intercepted by the block when placed on the smallest ball (or circle) would be greater than the number of lines intercepted by the block when placed on a bigger ball (or circle). As a matter of fact, the lines intercepted decrease in inverse proportion to the distance of the surface (or boundary) from the common center. Think of the lines as being representations of the path of photons.

From Figure 7.1 it is evident that the total number of lines that pass through the first circle also pass through the second and the third and the fourth and so on. This interception also occurs with three-dimensional objects. In this case the surface area of a sphere—such as a golf ball, tennis ball, or bowling ball—is proportional to the square of the radius:

$$\text{Surface area of sphere (A)} \propto \text{radius squared } (r^2) \qquad (7.1)$$

Thus, the number of lines (which represent photons) per unit surface of the golf ball is proportional to the total number of lines divided by the radius of the golf ball squared:

$$\begin{array}{c}\text{Number of lines per}\\ \text{unit surface area of}\\ \text{golf ball}\end{array} \propto \frac{\text{Total number of lines}}{r^2 \text{ golf ball}} \qquad (7.2)$$

The same rule obtains for the number of lines per unit surface area on the basketball:

$$\begin{array}{c}\text{Number of lines per}\\ \text{unit surface area of}\\ \text{basketball}\end{array} \propto \frac{\text{Total number of lines}}{r^2 \text{ basketball}} \qquad (7.3)$$

Since the surface area of the basketball is larger, in that it has a much larger radius than the golf ball, and the total number of lines remains the same, the basketball must have fewer lines per unit surface area than the golf ball. Notice that the inverse square of the radius is used in the preceding calculation—thus the origin of the term, "inverse square law."

To express this relationship quantitatively, the following convention is employed. The source of photons is treated as a point source located at the center of the sphere. In general, for reasonable distances and source sizes, this approximation is adequate. Then a reference point is picked: one unit distance away. This unit distance can be 1 meter, 1 centimeter, 1 inch, 1 foot—whatever is the most convenient unit to use. In this text, 1 meter has been chosen for consistency. As a result, knowing the number of photons at a distance of 1 meter (or any other unit distance) from the source, the number of photons at any other distance can be obtained, as follows:

$$\begin{array}{c}\text{Number of photons}\\ \text{at 1 m}\\ \text{(unit distance)}\end{array} \cdot (1\ \text{m})^2 = \begin{array}{c}\text{Number of photons}\\ \text{elsewhere}\end{array} \cdot \begin{array}{c}(\text{distance})^2\\ \text{in meters}\\ \text{from source}\end{array} \quad (7.4)$$

Example 7.1

A source of photons, as measured at a distance of 1 meter, emits 1000 photons. How many photons will be measured at a distance of 5 meters?

$$1000\ \text{photons} \cdot (1\ \text{m})^2 = \text{x photons} \cdot (5\ \text{m})^2$$

$$\frac{1000\ \text{photons}}{25\ \text{m}^2} \cdot 1\ \text{m}^2 = \text{x}$$

$$40\ \text{photons} = \text{x}$$

Two things are worth noting in the previous example. The first is the tremendous decrease in the number of photons encountered by the measuring unit, which could be the technician or physician himself. From 1000 photons measured at 1 meter, only 40 are measured at a distance five times as far from the source. This reduction in exposure is impressive. In fact, distance is the most effective means of protection against photons because it is unrelated to either the energy or source of photons. So safety can be purely a function of being far enough away.

The second item worthy of note is that, since the distance units cancel out, any unit distance will do as a reference. It does not matter whether the number of photons is measured at 1 centimeter or at 1 meter so long as both the reference distance and the distance of interest are measured in the *same* units.

Finally, this last observation means that, if the number of photons is known at *any* distance from the source, the number of photons that would be measured at any other distance can be calculated using the same simple rule:

$$\begin{array}{c}\text{Number of photons}\\ \text{at particular}\\ \text{distance from source}\end{array} \cdot (\text{distance})^2 = \begin{array}{c}\text{Number of photons}\\ \text{at any distance}\end{array} \cdot (\text{distance})^2 \quad (7.5)$$

Example 7.2

If 2000 photons are measured at a distance of 4 meters from a source, how many photons will be measured at a distance of 8 meters?

$$2000 \text{ photons} \cdot (4 \text{ m})^2 = x \text{ photons} \cdot (8 \text{ m})^2$$

$$\frac{2000 \text{ photons} \cdot 16 \text{ m}^2}{64 \text{ m}^2} = x$$

$$500 \text{ photons} = x$$

In the preceding example, although the distance from the photon source doubled, i.e., changed by a factor of 2 ($2 \times 4 = 8$), the number of photons measured decreased by a factor of 2^2, or 4. If the distance had changed by a factor of 3, for example, from 4 to 12 meters ($3 \times 4 = 12$), the number of photons would have decreased by 3^2, or 9. This example emphasizes again that distance is the best protection against photons. In fact, distance is the best protection against all kinds of ionizing radiation. Charged particles have a very short range (distance of travel), even in air, and neutrons have a small penetrating power when compared to that of photons.

In conclusion, put as much distance between a person and a source of ionizing radiation as possible. However, no amount of distance completely eliminates all photons; rather, distance helps reduce the number of photons encountered to an acceptable, or miniscule, level.

In practical terms, x-ray technicians and physicians should be as far away as possible when the x-ray tube is energized. Nuclear medicine technicians and physicians should stand as far away as possible from a patient injected with radioactive material. A good idea is to position the patient as quickly and efficiently as possible; then while the image is being taken, move away, however, always taking patient safety into consideration.

SHIELDING

The third and last type of protection against ionizing radiation consists of placing a barrier, or shield, between the radiation and the rest of the world. This barrier takes many different forms.

To shield from alpha particles, a thin sheet of paper is generally sufficient. For beta particles having those energies common in the radiologic and health sciences, a few millimeters of aluminum or a similar material is sufficient. When dealing with photons, the problem is not so simple. As with distance, no amount of shielding eliminates all photons. In addition, shielding has inherent problems in terms of weight and cost. It is only practical to surround a source of ionizing radiation with so much shielding—as in transporting a radionuclide —before it can be moved only with a forklift. Equally, an x-ray machine can be surrounded by just so much shielding before the cost of building the containing wall becomes prohibitive. For these reasons, the MPD is used to set standards of exposure; then distance and shielding are used together to meet these standards.

Half-Value Layer

To calculate the amount of shielding required, a concept known as the half-value layer (HVL) is used. This concept applies only in the case of photons.

If a beam of photons consists of only a single energy, the beam is referred to as monoenergetic. A beam of photons may be composed of many energies, generally the case with x-rays. As a result, it is common to speak of quality and quantity of a beam of photons.

Quality refers to the energy of particular photons, and quantity refers to the number of photons that has each specific energy. Quality and quantity are described together in a concept known as intensity, defined as the total energy contained in the beam (quality × quantity) per unit area per unit time.

$$\text{I (intensity)} = \frac{\text{E total}}{\text{Area} \cdot \text{Time}} \tag{7.6}$$

The area referred to is the cross-sectional area of the beam at a particular point in space. Since most beams of photons spread out as they move away from the source, it is important to specify where the intensity is being calculated.

In the following discussion of HVL, a monoenergetic beam of photons has been assumed. The application to a non-monoenergetic (polyenergetic) beam is made afterward.

Consider a beam of photons approaching a barrier, e.g., a simple wall, as shown in Figure 7.2. Some of the photons penetrate to the far side of the wall, and some are attenuated by the wall material. The number of photons absorbed by the wall is a function of both the energy of the photons and the atomic

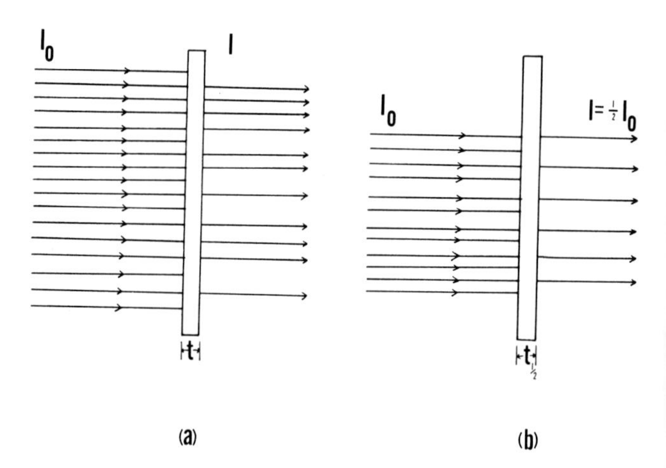

Figure 7.2: Half-Value Layer (HVL): (a) A barrier of thickness "t" stops a number of photons consistent with the linear attenuation coefficient μ. (b) Consistent with the linear attenuation coefficient μ of the barrier, a thickness "$t_{\frac{1}{2}}$" is chosen such that half of the photons are attenuated out of the original beam.

number and density of the material composing the wall. In general, two principles apply:

1. The more energetic the photons, the less likely they are to be attenuated.
2. The smaller the atomic number and the less dense the material composing the barrier, the less likely it is to attenuate the photons.

The relationship between the number and energy of photons penetrating the barrier and the material and thickness of the barrier is expressed as follows:

$$N = N_o\, e^{-\mu t} \qquad (7.7)$$

N_o represents the number of photons arriving at the barrier, N represents the number of photons leaving the barrier, t represents thickness of the barrier, and μ is a constant that characterizes the ability of the barrier material to attenuate photons of that particular energy. The constant μ is commonly called the *linear attenuation coefficient*. It is important to remember that μ depends not only on the barrier material but also on the energy of photons. The value of μ can be obtained using equation 7.7. An example follows.

Example 7.3

A beam of 5000 monoenergetic photons is reduced to 3000 photons by a barrier consisting of a slab of tin 1.0 centimeter thick. What is the linear attenuation coefficient of the tin slab for these photons?

$$N = N_o\, e^{-\mu t}$$

$$3000 = 5000\, e^{-\mu(1\ \text{cm})}$$

$$\frac{3000}{5000} = e^{-\mu(1\ \text{cm})} = \frac{1}{e^{\mu(1\ \text{cm})}}$$

Inverting the preceding expression:

$$\frac{5}{3} = e^{\mu(1\ \text{cm})}$$

Taking the natural logarithm of both sides (a brief review of logs is given in Appendix III):

$$\ln \frac{5}{3} = \mu(1 \text{ cm})$$

From Table III.1:

$$0.05827 = \mu(1 \text{ cm})$$

$$\frac{0.05827}{\text{cm}} = \mu$$

or

$$0.05827 \text{ cm}^{-1} = \mu$$

From this computation it can be seen that μ is measured in units of reciprocal length.

When the thickness t of the barrier is chosen such that the original number of photons N_0 is reduced to one-half of its value, $N = \frac{1}{2}N_0$, then t is written as $t_{1/2}$ and is referred to as the HVL.

$$N = \tfrac{1}{2}N_0 = N_0 e^{-\mu t_{1/2}} \qquad (7.8)$$

The HVL—or, as it is sometimes called, the half-value thickness (HVT)—is a measure of the quality or penetrating power of the beam. The higher the energy of the photons, the thicker will be the HVL.

Using equation 7.8, a useful relation can be derived between μ and $t_{1/2}$:

$$\tfrac{1}{2}N_0 = N_0 e^{-\mu t_{1/2}}$$

Divide both sides by N_0:

$$\tfrac{1}{2} = e^{-\mu t_{1/2}}$$

Take the natural logarithm of both sides:

$$\ln(\tfrac{1}{2}) = -\mu t_{1/2}$$

$$\ln 1 - \ln 2 = -\mu t_{1/2}$$

Since

$$\ln 1 = 0$$

$$-\ln 2 = -\mu t_{1/2}$$

Multiply both sides by minus one:

$$\ln 2 = \mu t_{1/2} \tag{7.9}$$

This result gives two relations. (1) Divide both sides of equation 7.9 by μ:

$$\frac{\ln 2}{\mu} = t_{1/2} \tag{7.10}$$

or (2) divide both sides of equation 7.9 by $t_{1/2}$:

$$\frac{\ln 2}{t_{1/2}} = \mu \tag{7.11}$$

Equation 7.10 says that, if μ is known for a particular barrier, the thickness of the HVL can be determined. If, on the other hand, the thickness of the HVL is known or determined experimentally, the value of μ can be calculated.

The concept of HVL can now be used to determine how much shielding is needed in any practical application. Consider equation 7.7:

$$N = N_0 e^{-\mu t}$$

Divide both sides by N_0:

$$\frac{N}{N_0} = e^{-\mu t}$$

Use equation 7.11 and substitute in the value of μ:

$$\frac{N}{N_0} = e^{\frac{-\ln 2}{t_{1/2}} \cdot t}$$

Using the properties of logs:

$$\frac{N}{N_0} = e^{-\ln 2 \; t/t_{1/2}}$$

Since ln 1 = 0, one can write:

$$\frac{N}{N_0} = e^{\ln 1 - \ln 2^{t/t_{1/2}}}$$

$$= \frac{1}{e^{\ln 2^{t/t_{1/2}}}}$$

Finally, because $e^{\ln Z} = Z$, one obtains:

$$\frac{N}{N_0} = \frac{1}{2^{t/t_{1/2}}} \qquad (7.12)$$

This equation says that, if the ratio of N to N_0 is known, the number of HVL's needed to produce that ratio can be determined. It is more useful to write equation 7.12 in inverted form:

$$\frac{N_0}{N} = 2^{t/t_{1/2}} \qquad (7.13)$$

When the thickness of barrier t is divided by the thickness of an HVL, $t_{1/2}$, the number of HVL's needed is obtained. The original number of photons divided by the number of photons to which the beam is to be reduced then gives two raised to the number of HVL's needed. This result simplifies matters consid-

Table 7.1

The Powers of 2

n	2^n	$\frac{1}{2^n}$
0	1	1.0
1	2	0.5
2	4	0.25
3	8	0.125
4	16	0.0625
5	32	0.03125
6	64	0.015625
7	128	0.0078125
8	256	0.0039062
9	512	0.0019531
10	1,024	0.0009765

erably because it is easy to remember the powers of two, which are given in Table 7.1 up to 2^{10}. To obtain any entry in the table, just take the number before it and multiply by two. A practical example of the use of equation 7.13 follows.

Example 7.4

It is necessary to reduce a source of 5000 monoenergetic photons to 1000 photons. How many HVL's of a particular substance are needed?

$$\frac{N_0}{N} = 2^{t/t_{1/2}} \quad (7.13)$$

$$\frac{5000}{1000} = 2^{t/t_{1/2}}$$

Hence

$$5 = 2^{t/t_{1/2}}$$

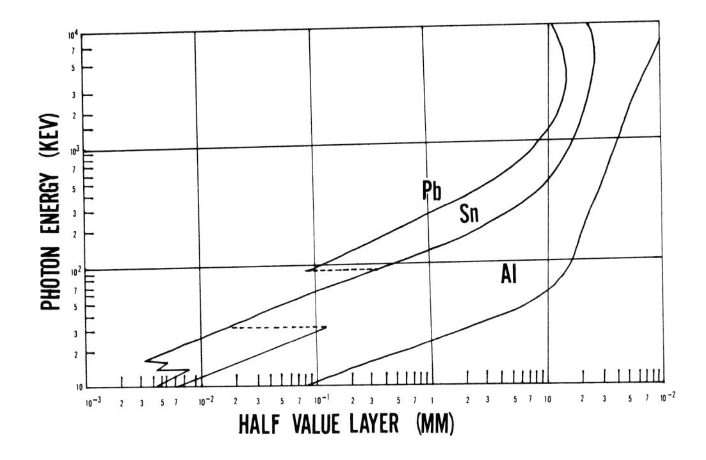

Figure 7.3: Half-Value Layers for Photons 10 keV to 10 MeV: One curve is for lead (Pb), one for tin (Sn), and one for aluminum (Al). Curves prepared by G.L. Rhinehart and N.F. Modine, National Center for Radiological Health, U.S. Public Health Service; reproduced with permission of the U.S. Department of Health, Education and Welfare, Public Health Service, Food and Drug Administration, Bureau of Radiological Health, from the Radiological Health Handbook. rev. ed., January, 1970.

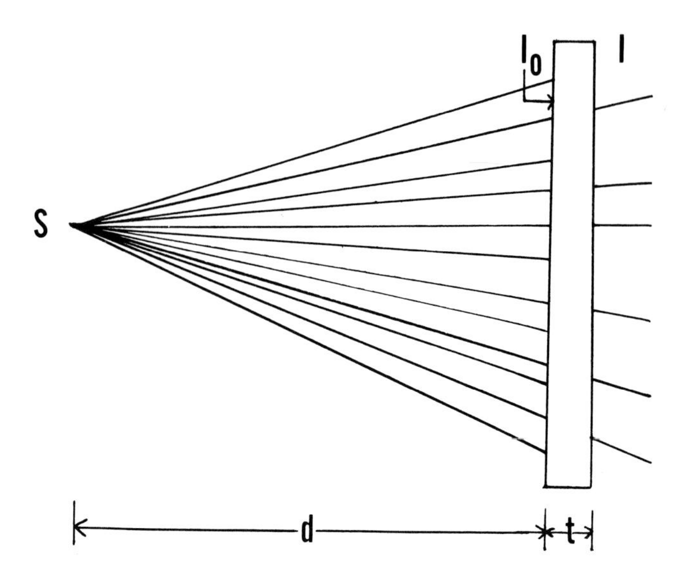

Figure 7.4: Distance and shielding used together to reduce the intensity from the photon source (S).

From Table 7.1, 5 is between 2 and 3 HVL's. Hence, a little more than 2 HVL's of material is needed to reduce the photon number to the desired value. The actual thickness of HVL is determined by the photon energy and the barrier material. Figure 7.3 gives a graph of HVL's for different materials and photon energies.

In the beginning of this section it was mentioned that distance is often used in conjunction with shielding. Figure 7.4 shows how distance and shielding can be simultaneously used to reduce the photon number to some designated level.

Example 7.5

A monoenergetic source of photons emits 5000 photons as measured at a distance of 1.0 meter. A barrier is placed 5.0 meters away. It is necessary to reduce the number of photons to 10. How many HVL's thick should the barrier be?

First, the number of photons N_0 arriving at the barrier must be found from equation 7.3:

$$5000 \cdot (1\ \text{m})^2 = x \cdot (5\ \text{m})^2$$

$$\frac{5000\ \text{m}^2}{25\ \text{m}^2} = 200 = N_o$$

Now use equation 7.13 to obtain:

$$\frac{N_o}{N} = 2^{t/t_{1/2}}$$

$$\frac{200}{10} = 2^{t/t_{1/2}}$$

$$20 = 2^{t/t_{1/2}}$$

From Table 7.1 it is evident that a barrier thickness of between 4 and 5 HVL's is needed.

Polyenergetic Beams of Photons

Last, it is necessary to look at the characteristics of polyenergetic beams of photons. When a beam of photons contains more than one energy, photons that have the least energy are usually stopped first. The weeding out of these lower-energy, "soft," photons changes the quality of the beam; in fact, the beam contains photons that have a higher average energy. This phenomenon is known as beam hardening. Since the lower-energy photons are the first to be stopped, the first HVL of shielding is thin because these photons are relatively easy to stop. As the beam is hardened, more shielding is needed to reduce the number of photons in the beam to one-half. Hence, in a polyenergetic beam of photons, the HVL thicknesses increase as the beam is hardened. Each HVL thickness must be calculated separately. For a close approximation, calculate the intensity of the beam I_o entering the barrier instead of the number of photons in the beam. This intensity value is based on the average energy of the beam.*

*Generally speaking, a combination of three metallic filters is placed in front of the anode of the x-ray tube. These filters serve to harden the beam and raise its average energy closer to the peak kilovoltage value, thereby preventing the more harmful soft x-rays from reaching the patient. Aluminum alloy filters are often used because they are efficient in removing soft x-rays.

In summary, no one method of radiation protection is entirely effective. A radiation worker must be aware of each method and must take best advantage of each. Awareness of and a healthy respect for danger associated with ionizing radiation are the first steps toward formulating a personal protection plan. Next must be a commitment to the principle, "the best exposure is no exposure." Then comes a firm resolution to adopt and use a personal protection plan. Finally, a thorough knowledge of the principles of radiation protection enables a personal protection plan to become a practical reality.

BIBLIOGRAPHY

Hendee, W. R.: Interaction of x and gamma rays (Chapter 7). *In* Medical Radiation Physics. Chicago, Year Book Medical Publishers, 1970.

Johns, H. E., and Cunningham, J.R.: The absorption of radiation (Chapter 5). *In* The Physics of Radiology. Springfield, IL, Charles C Thomas, Publisher, 1974.

Radiological Health Handbook (rev. ed.). Rockville, MD, Department of Health, Education and Welfare, Public Health Service, U.S. Government Printing Office, Washington, D.C., January, 1970.

Protection from Radionuclides

section two

chapter 8

Good Working Habits

Wherever radionuclides are present, the principles of protection take on a twofold aspect: protection from external exposure and protection against internal exposure. A radionuclide present in a working area is outside the body and thus constitutes a potential external hazard. This radionuclide becomes an internal hazard when it is ingested, injected, absorbed through the skin, or inhaled.

COMMON EXTERNAL SOURCES OF RADIATION EXPOSURE

The most common source of external exposure is photons, and both radionuclides and x-ray machines are possible sources of photons. Radionuclides can be a source of beta and alpha particles as well.

Photons with energies greater than 100 keV are highly penetrating and can irradiate (expose) the entire body fairly uniformly. Photons that have smaller energies have less penetrating power and give a more superficial exposure, or dose, to the body. The exposure from low-energy photons is more localized in the sense that only a limited number of layers of skin or of skin plus other tissue may be exposed.

On the other hand, the external danger from alpha-emitting radionuclides is small. Even alpha particles with energies of up to 5 MeV would not be able to penetrate the dead outermost layers of the skin.

An external source of beta particles is a cause for more or less concern, depending upon the energy of the particles. Betas are very light when compared to alpha particles, but they do have charge. As a result of their light mass, they penetrate farther into any material than alpha particles do before losing their energy through ionization. Beta particles themselves can have a range in tissue up to 1.0 centimeter, but they rarely penetrate any farther into the human body than the outer layer of the skin. The more pressing danger from beta particles is associated with higher-energy particles.

As stated in Chapter 1, when high-energy electrons (a few keV and up) pass through matter, they are attracted, because of their negative charge, by the nuclei of the atoms of which the material is composed. This attraction deflects the electron from its path, and as a result, the electron radiates some energy in the form of a photon.

This process results in a slowing down of the electron, or a braking action, known commonly as bremsstrahlung. The heavy nuclei found in shielding materials, such as lead, have a greater probability of causing bremsstrahlung. Consequently, the container holding a radionuclide that is a pure beta emitter may be itself a source of photons.

PROTECTION FROM EXTERNAL SOURCES

To protect oneself from the external sources just described, the principles of time, distance, and shielding must be used. Unsealed radionuclides, particularly photon emitters, should be carefully stored in a lead container unit or behind lead bricks. It is normal to store small quantities of radionuclides, in either liquid or pill form, in individual vials, the vials then being placed inside small lead containers. These containers should in turn be placed in a lead-lined storage area, either into a large, heavily leaded container known as a pig or behind lead bricks.

When a vial is needed to administer a patient dose, it is taken from the pig or from behind the lead

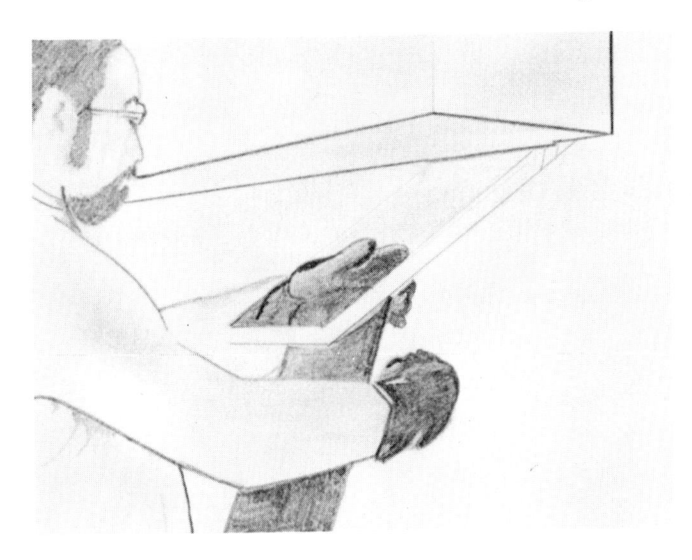

Figure 8.1: Lead glass shield for working with radionuclides.

bricks and the dose quickly withdrawn (or the pill removed). If the radionuclide is in liquid form, the dose is drawn up in a syringe. This syringe should have a lead glass liner around it, and it should be placed as quickly as possible into a lead container until the patient is injected. For the actual drawing up of doses, the facility should have a tabletop lead shield with a lead glass viewing area on top (Fig. 8.1). This type of shield protects the whole body of the radiation worker, even the sensitive lens of the eye, while still allowing a full visualization of the working area. If the hands are used directly, lead-lined gloves should be used. If these gloves are too awkward, plastic gloves should be used for purposes of isolation (as discussed later in this chapter). It is ideal to use a pair of tongs so that not even the hands are exposed. This consideration is an example of using the principles of shielding and distance together.

In laboratories or clinics where radionuclides are used, they should always be stored in a separate area. Wherever radionuclides are used, they should be shielded as well as practicable; the time of expo-

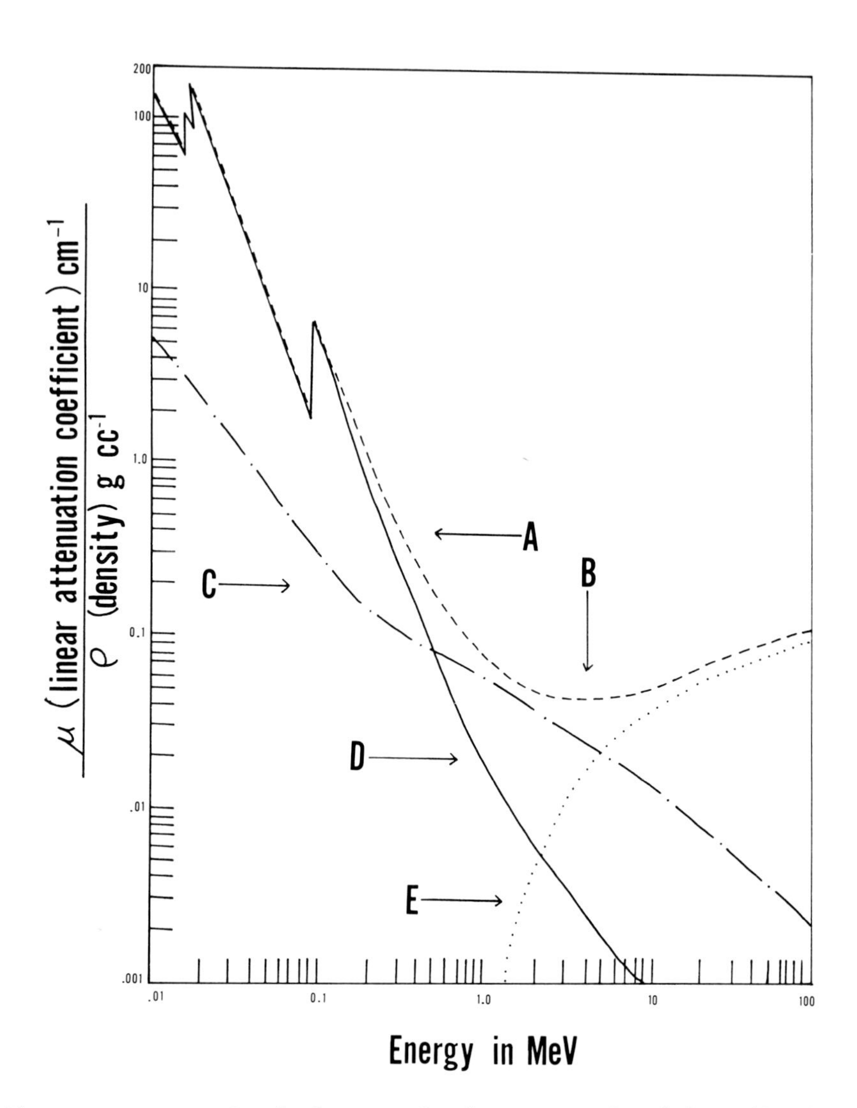

Figure 8.2: Graph showing the decrease in the ability of lead to attenuate photons whose energy is about 3 MeV. Note the decrease in the total attenuation coefficient (A) at B. C is the Compton scattering attenuation coefficient; D is the photoelectric attenuation coefficient; E is the pair production attenuation coefficient. All linear attenuation coefficients are divided by the density of lead. (Data obtained from G. R. White, NBS Report No. 1003 (1952); reproduced with permission of the U.S. Department of Health, Education and Welfare, Public Health Service, Food and Drug Administration, Bureau of Radiological Health, from the Radiological Health Handbook, rev. ed., January, 1970.)

sure should be reduced as much as possible by employing efficient working techniques; and tongs should be used along with other methods to increase the distance from the radionuclide.

A patient who has been given a photon-emitting radionuclide is also a source of external exposure. A radiation worker should be aware of this aspect and should position the patient as quickly as possible, then move away. Hovering over the patient unnecessarily only tends to increase the exposure. The patient should be cared for as meticulously as is appropriate, but the principles of time, distance, and shielding should also be applied. Some radiation workers may wish to wear a lead or tin apron. In some institutions lead or tin screens are placed near the patient while the study is being conducted.

Lead does have one peculiar property, which should be mentioned. A sharp drop in the ability of lead to attenuate or absorb photons occurs in the energy region of about 3 MeV. The reason for this drop is that in lead the probability for a photoelectric or a Compton interaction decreases rapidly as the photon energy approaches 3 MeV, and at the same time the probability for a pair-production interaction has not increased sufficiently. This characteristic of lead should be kept in mind when shielding is designed for photon sources, such as high-energy radiation therapy machines or high-energy radionuclides. Figure 8.2 shows this phenomenon.

INTERNAL HAZARDS

The radiation worker must also take precautions against the hazards involved in the deposition of radionuclides within the body. Internal radioactive material produces continuous radiation exposure until it physically decays or is eliminated through normal metabolic processes. The control of internal radiation exposure, therefore, consists in preventing radionuclides from entering the body; hence, internal exposure control is essentially a problem of contamination control.

The amount of internal radiation exposure is a function of the type, energy, and amount of radionuclide inside the body. In addition, the internal hazard is dependent upon the size, shape, and biologic importance of the exposed organ within the body, and upon the length of time that the radionuclide remains there.

COMMON INTERNAL SOURCES OF RADIATION EXPOSURE

Alpha particles, because of their large mass and double positive charge, have a very short range both in air and in tissue. The range of alpha particles, even with energies as high as 4 to 9 MeV, is only a few hundredths of a millimeter in tissue and a few hundredths of a centimeter in air. Alpha particles are highly ionizing, and since their range is short, all this energy is deposited in a very small region near where the alpha particle is emitted. Further, the RBE of alpha particles for tissue is considerably greater (about 20 times) than that of photons or beta particles.

In short, while alpha particles pose no serious external threat, when deposited throughout a vital organ, they can cause considerable damage. What is more, many alpha-emitting radionuclides concentrate in tissues like compact and trabecular bone, usually on the surface. Bone has an organic component and a mineral matrix. The turnover rate is different for each. Thus, depending on where the alpha emitter concentrates, the activity could decrease only as fast as the physical bone tissue turnover. As a result, a radionuclide that is an alpha emitter can still cause damage long after it has been admitted to the body. For these reasons, long-lived alpha emitters are poor agents for diagnostic purposes.

Beta particles, because they are much lighter than alpha particles and are singly charged, have a larger range in both air and tissue and are 20 times less destructive; however, beta particles are ionizing particles, and rarely is their range long enough for them to leave the organ in which they are produced.

As a result, they deposit all or most of their energy in that organ. Should this organ be a vital one and should the quantity of beta emitters in the organ be large, serious consequences could result.

One example of a possibly dangerous beta emitter is strontium-90 (^{90}Sr), which has a physical half-life of 27.4 years. This radionuclide is produced in fission reactions, and large quantities of it have been observed in the radioactive fallout following nuclear bomb testing. The nuclide that results from the beta decay of ^{90}Sr—namely, yttrium-90 (^{90}Y)—is also a beta emitter. Strontium is a bone seeker and this factor, coupled with its long physical half-life, makes it an undesirable internal radionuclide. So far, the total dose contaminant to the entire world population from ^{90}Sr fallout has been less than 100 Gy.

A second example is ^{131}I. This radionuclide is commonly used in nuclear medicine because iodine is a thyroid seeker. It is, however, both a beta and a gamma emitter. The physical half-life (defined in Chapter 10) of ^{131}I is approximately 8 days. This half-life, together with the high metabolic rate of the thyroid gland, makes ^{131}I less of a hazard than, say, ^{90}Sr; but the probability of a person who works in the radiologic and health sciences encountering ^{131}I is great.

Photons, because of their relatively low ability to ionize, deposit much less energy per unit path length in tissue than do either alpha or beta particles. Radionuclides that emit alpha and/or beta particles generally emit photons as well. In that case, most of the absorbed dose is due to the particulate radiation, and not much is attributable to the photons. For this reason, radionuclides that are pure photon emitters represent much less of an internal hazard than do either alpha or beta emitters.

COMMON METHODS OF INTERNAL ENTRY

The three common methods of unintentional internal acquisition of radionuclides are inhalation, ingestion, or absorption. When radionuclides are intentionally administered internally, they generally enter the body by injection, inhalation, or ingestion. Here, only the unintentional aspects of entry to the body are discussed.

Inhalation

Inhalation of airborne materials is a serious internal hazard. The absorption, retention, and elimination of material taken into the lungs depend on such things as the size of the particle inhaled, its solubility, and the rate of respiration of the individual inhaling it. Persons should particularly guard against inhaling radionuclides in the form of powders or volatile liquids. Iodine is a particularly volatile liquid, and radioactive isotopes of iodine in liquid form are frequently used in chemical laboratory tests (in vitro) as well as in diagnostic tests and therapeutic treatments (in vivo) where they are administered directly to patients.

Consequently, whenever volatile liquids are stored or used, a chemical fume hood should be used. The inner surfaces of this hood should be made of a nonporous material, such as stainless steel, or be covered with a strippable paint to permit easy decontamination. A fume hood that vents radioactive materials must have its output strictly regulated. The amount of radioactivity allowed per cubic centimeter is given for some selected radionuclides in Table 8.1. Rarely are such quantities a problem, except in case of accidents.

As an alternative to a fume hood, a totally enclosed chamber, known as a glove box, may be used. The advantages of a glove box are not only that it confines any contamination within a totally enclosed space but also that it uses a very small air supply to prevent the escape of activity into the working atmosphere when compared to the generous airflow necessary in the usual hood system. Among the disadvantages are the extra time and labor involved and the difficulties of working inside the box, as well as those associated with removing the radionuclide from the glove box. On the other hand, glove boxes are indispensable for working

Table 8.1

Maximum Permissible Concentrations of Radionuclides in Air and Water

Radio-nuclide	Unrestricted Areas				Restricted Areas (40-hour week)			
	Water		Air		Water		Air	
	$Bqcc^{-1}$	$(pCicc^{-1})$	$Bqcc^{-1}$	$(pCicc^{-1})$	$Bqcc^{-1}$	$(pCicc^{-1})$	$Bqcc^{-1}$	$(pCicc^{-1})$
^{14}C	2.95	(80.0)	$3.7 \cdot 10^{-3}$	(0.1)	$7.4 \cdot 10^{2}$	$(2 \cdot 10^{4})$	0.148	(4.0)
^{3}H	111	$(3 \cdot 10^{3})$	$7.4 \cdot 10^{-3}$	(0.2)	$3.7 \cdot 10^{3}$	$(1 \cdot 10^{5})$	0.185	(5.0)
^{131}I	$1.11 \cdot 10^{-4}$	(0.3)	$3.7 \cdot 10^{-6}$	$(1 \cdot 10^{-4})$	2.22	(60)	$3.33 \cdot 10^{-4}$	(0.009)
^{125}I	$7.4 \cdot 10^{-3}$	(0.2)	$2.96 \cdot 10^{-6}$	$(8 \cdot 10^{-5})$	1.48	(40)	$1.85 \cdot 10^{-4}$	(0.005)
^{32}P	0.74	(20.0)	$7.4 \cdot 10^{-5}$	$(2 \cdot 10^{-3})$	18.5	$(5 \cdot 10^{2})$	$2.59 \cdot 10^{-3}$	(0.07)
^{51}Cr	7.4	(200.0)	$2.96 \cdot 10^{-3}$	$(8 \cdot 10^{-2})$	$1.85 \cdot 10^{3}$	$(5 \cdot 10^{4})$	$7.4 \cdot 10^{-2}$	(2.0)
^{133}Xe	—		$1.11 \cdot 10^{-3}$	(0.3)	—		0.37	(10)

Taken from the U.S. Code of Federal Regulations, Title 10, Part 20, as of December, 1969.

with dry powders and are highly recommended for work with alpha emitters and low-energy beta emitters such as tritium.

It is likewise desirable that all equipment needed for the handling of radioactive material be segregated and used only for this work. One method of accomplishing this objective is to tag the various items used as "radioactive materials." It is particularly important to tag small items such as glassware and handling equipment such as tongs, which can easily transfer contamination from fume hoods to the open laboratory.

Ingestion

Ingested material can enter the body by absorption from the gastrointestinal (GI) tract. The chemical and physical form of the ingested material determines the percent that is absorbed by the bloodstream. A large proportion of insoluble ingested material is rapidly excreted in normal body wastes. A significant enough internal hazard may be caused simply by the irradiation of the gastrointestinal tract itself.

It is good radiation-protection practice never to take unessential personal items into the active area. All food, drink, smoking materials, and cosmetics should remain outside the working area, including the scanning rooms; and nothing should be placed in the mouth while working in an active area. This practice is essential when potentially contaminated equipment is used. Such equipment should never be handled with bare hands. In particular, pipettes should never be operated by mouth suction. Any type of glassmaking in active areas or on contaminated equipment should be done with special techniques that avoid forming the glass by blowing with the mouth.

Absorption

Absorption through unbroken skin or through abrasions, cuts, and punctures is still another way that unwanted radioactive material may enter the bloodstream. To prevent this type of entry, all personnel working with radionuclides should follow proper procedures and wear protective clothing, particularly gloves, to prevent contact between radionuclides and the skin. Patients who have received an internal dose of a radionuclide often excrete some of this material in their sweat. It is, therefore, important that the radiation worker wear gloves not only when handling the radionuclides but also when attending to radioactive patients, particularly when doing a brain scan because pertechnetate goes readily to the sweat glands.

In this same vein, all personnel working in radiation areas must wear proper protective clothing. The clothing change considered necessary depends on the level of activity and the types of procedure performed. In ordinary tracer laboratories, a standard laboratory coat is sufficient. In intermediate-level laboratories, such as a radiation oncology laboratory, laboratory coats and a change of shoes may be compulsory; or a complete change of clothing plus a shoe change may be required.

CONTAMINATION CONTROL

Internal exposure control is exercised by preventing the entry of radioactive material into the body. Essentially the problem is to control contamination. Two of the fundamental principles of such control are containment and cleanliness.

Containment is that form of radioactive contamination control which seeks to restrict radioactive materials to specified areas. The choice of operating techniques for handling radioactive materials is an important part of achieving containment goals. For instance, when working with radionuclides in liquid form, the working surface should be covered by either plastic trays or a layer of disposable absorbent material to soak up spills. Materials used extensively include blotting paper and diaper paper, which is heavy absorbent paper backed with an impervious material such as oiled paper. The latter is preferable because it prevents liquids from ever reaching the bench top.

Second, when introducing a new procedure, try it several times with inactive materials before undertaking any manipulations involving radionuclides. Unexpected difficulties are uncovered in this way, and equipment weaknesses detected. Procedural modifications can be made as necessary.

Third, single containers should never be used. Instead use suitable trays or double containers that are capable of holding the primary containers entirely.

Cleanliness and good housekeeping are the most effective supplements to proper operating techniques. These practices not only minimize the spread of contamination but also prevent the build-up of significant levels of contamination.

Cleanliness is not just associated with visible good housekeeping; it also assumes a regular monitoring of the laboratory and of the personnel followed by prompt decontamination when necessary. Working surfaces and floors should be checked regularly. Portable survey instruments are sufficient to monitor bench surfaces and floors where no sources of sufficient strength to cause a high room background are stored. The survey instrument chosen should be one that has the proper response for the type and energy of radiation being used. End-window G-M tubes are the most commonly used instruments for this type of monitoring.

If a sufficiently high background exists, or if low-energy beta emitters like tritium or low-energy photon emitters like ^{125}I are involved, the detection of traces of contamination with a survey instrument is difficult. In this case, surfaces are wiped with small pieces of filter paper or other suitable material. These wipes are then removed and counted with an appropriate counter; ideally, a well counter or a liquid scintillation counter is used. In any case, the counter selected must have a detector that is sensitive to the type and energy of the radiation involved.

It is good practice to have everyone working with radionuclides wash and monitor his hands

Table 8.2

Maximum Permissible Body Burdens for Occupationally Exposed Personnel

Radio-nuclide	Total Body Burden MBq	(mCi)	Critical Organ Burden MBq	(mCi)	Critical Organ
^{14}C	14.8	(0.4)	11.1	(0.3)	Fat
^{3}H	74.0	(2.0)	37.0	(1.0)	Body tissue
^{131}I	1.84	(0.05)	$2.59 \cdot 10^{-2}$	$(0.7 \cdot 10^{-3})$	Thyroid
^{32}P	1.11	(0.03)	0.222	(0.006)	Bone
^{51}Cr	2.95	(0.8)	37.0	(1.0)	Lung

Reproduced with permission of the U.S. Department of Health, Education and Welfare, Public Health Service, Food and Drug Administration, Bureau of Radiological Health, from the Radiological Health Handbook, rev. ed., 1970.

Taken from National Bureau of Standards Handbook 69, U.S. Government Printing Office, Washington, DC, 1963.

Also see ICRP, Report No. 17, Protection of Patients in Radionuclide Investigations. Elmsford, NY, Pergamon Press, Ltd., 1971.

Also see NCRP Publication No. 22, 1959, and Addendum, 1963.

before leaving the area to eat. Radiation workers should be checked regularly by some sort of whole-body counting method to determine their internal radiation body burden. Keep in mind that the allowable internal body burden is different for different radionuclides. The maximum permissible body burdens for some radionuclides are summarized in Table 8.2.

MANAGEMENT OF ACCIDENTS

In the event of an accident involving the contamination of an area, personnel protection and the immediate confinement of the contamination are of primary importance. A standardized approach should be well known and followed by all personnel in the laboratory or clinic. Emergency procedures should be posted in each area along with the person, usually the radiation protection officer (RPO), to be contacted in case of an accident involving radiation. A typical plan follows.

Confinement

The spread of contamination should be prevented by

1. closing doors and windows.
2. turning off fans, air conditioners, and other ventilation if possible.
3. closing ventilation ducts if possible.
4. vacating the room but not the area, so as not to spread the contamination; in case of a liquid spill, leaving shoes and other garments at the door.
5. locking the door and, if airborne material is involved, sealing edges with tape.

Once confinement has been accomplished, the cleanup can be conducted later. A well-constructed plan might be as follows.

Decontamination

A specific plan must be worked out considering the physical facilities and the properties of the contaminating materials. Such a plan should include:

1. monitoring the contaminated area to determine the extent of contamination and the hazard.
2. making sure the decontamination personnel wear sufficient protective clothing.
3. in the case of liquid spills, proceeding with decontamination by scrubbing surfaces with a detergent solution, always working toward the center of the contaminated area, taking care not to spread the contamination to less active areas.

During the decontamination procedure, frequent and thorough monitoring, especially of all personnel and materials, should be performed before either is permitted to move into clean (uncontaminated) areas.

PERSONNEL DECONTAMINATION

When a radiation worker or a patient becomes or suspects that he is contaminated, certain measures should be taken immediately. A G-M tube or other suitable detector of high sensitivity should be used to locate the area of contamination. Any contaminated clothing, including shoes, should be immediately removed and placed in a lead-shielded storage area until it has decayed to a safe level—usually 7 to 10 half-lives of the radionuclide spilled.

When the hands or other body surfaces have become contaminated, care must be taken to prevent the spread of the radioactive material to other areas, especially to open wounds. Loose particles of contamination should be immediately removed. Decontamination methods that spread localized material or increase penetration of the skin should be avoided.

Decontamination of wounds should be accomplished under the supervision of a physician when possible. An effective method is to irrigate the wound(s) profusely with tepid water and to scrub gently with a soft brush, if necessary. It is important to avoid the use of hot water, which increases the blood flow to the skin surface; or of highly alkaline soap, which may fixate the contaminant; or of organic solvents, which may increase skin penetration by the contaminant.

For intact skin, the decontamination rules are similar. Wet the skin thoroughly and apply detergent. Work up a full lather, and keep it wet. Work the lather into the contaminated area by rubbing gently for an extended period, at least 3 minutes, while at the same time tepid-to-cold water is frequently applied. Rinse the area thoroughly with tepid-to-cold water, trying to limit run-off water to the contaminated areas. In the case of the fingers and toes, if monitoring shows excess radioactivity at the tips, it will help to clip the appropriate nails. If monitoring continues to show that the intact skin areas are highly radioactive, wash again, scrubbing with a soft brush, if necessary. If the radiation level still persists, help should be sought from someone knowledgeable in the area of radiation protection.

BIBLIOGRAPHY

Shapiro, J.: Practical aspects of the use of radionuclides Part V. *In* Radiation Protection. Cambridge, MA, Harvard University Press, 1972.

Simmons, G. H., and Alexander, G. W.: Principles of radiation protection (Chapter XV). *In* A Training Manual for Nuclear Medicine Technologists. Rockville, MD, U.S. Department of Health, Education and Welfare, Public Health Service, Bureau of Radiological Health, October, 1970.

chapter 9

RADIONUCLIDES AND THE LAW

The production, transportation, possession, and use of radionuclides are strictly regulated by law. This regulation is an effort by society to prevent radiation accidents and to ensure proper corrective procedures should such accidents occur. So a strict licensing system controls the different phases of activity associated with radionuclides. These licenses are issued at federal, state, or local levels, depending upon a number of different factors. In general, these licenses include regulations that require a certain amount of expertise on the part of the recipient and some record keeping. In the radiologic and health sciences, the technical and administrative measures involved in complying with the law are relatively minor. Nevertheless, they should be attended to with care, diligence, and perseverance.

LICENSING

Through the Atomic Energy Act of 1954, Congress authorized the federal government to control reactor-produced (i.e., fission-produced) radionuclides, usually referred to as by-product material. This act provided for programs to develop use of atomic energy for the general welfare and also to regulate its use to protect public health and safety.

Nuclear Regulatory Commission

The regulatory power created by this act, with respect to fissile products, is vested in the Nuclear Regulatory Commission (NRC), formerly the Atomic Energy Commission (AEC). The Code of Federal Regulations (CFR) is that set of laws enacted by federal agencies empowered by Congress to make regulations. Title 10 of the CFR pertains to atomic energy. The most important sections for radionuclide users are:

1. Standards for Protection Against Radiation (Part 20).
2. Rules of General Applicability to Licensing of By-product Material (Part 30).
3. Human Uses of By-product Material (Part 35).

Radionuclides that are not reactor-produced, such as radium, or those that are produced in a cyclotron, such as ^{123}I, are not regulated by the NRC. However, if reactor-produced radionuclides are being used along with other sources of radiation, the NRC may review all radiation work. The reasoning is that the agency is responsible for determining that the user has complied with exposure standards for the use of reactor-produced radionuclides when added to exposure from all other radiation sources. The regulation of all radionuclides that are not reactor-produced is incorporated into state or other health codes, such as those of the military. The disadvantage is that the formulating of regulations is then under executive, rather than legislative, control.

What is more, as mentioned in Chapter 6, in certain instances the NRC has entered into agreements with certain states such that the states themselves regulate fission products as well. In these cases state regulations may be more, but must not be less, stringent than those of the NRC. In turn, states may enter into agreements with certain city or local governments to allow local regulation of radionuclides. Again, the same rule of more, but not less, stringent regulations applies. An example of a state entering into agreement with one of its cities is that of the State of New York and New York City.

Radiation Control Health and Safety Act of 1968

It is well to note that radionuclides have been strictly regulated since they became available in a practicable manner following World War II. The same is not true of x-rays or of other types of radiation because their use became very widespread before their possible harmful effects became known. The Radiation Control Health and Safety Act of 1968 was the first piece of legislation regulating x-rays, microwaves, and other radiation emissions from electronic products. In this Act, Congress directed that the Department of Health, Education and Welfare develop and administer performance standards to control the emission of radiation from electronic products such as microwave ovens and color TV sets. It also authorized research by public and private organizations into the effects and control of such radiation emissions. This regulation is usually done through the Bureau of Radiological Health. Unfortunately, the implementation of this Act has been hampered by many industrial concerns and "grandfather" clauses, but at least safety standards have been established and publicized. Enforcement is difficult, but when a worker's safety is involved, sometimes the Department of Labor, which enforces the Occupational Health and Safety Act (OHSA) (Title 29 of the CFR), can be of help.

Authorization

When a program of work with radionuclides is initiated, authorization must be obtained from the appropriate government agency, usually the NRC. This commission has decided that all radionuclides produced in reactors can be obtained and used only under specific or general NRC licenses. Certain exceptions may be made in terms of particular items, concentrations, and quantities. These exceptions rarely apply to any work that would be performed in the radiologic and health sciences and so are not listed here.

A specific license is issued to a named applicant after the commission has reviewed and approved the proposer's application. This application must include the proposed radionuclides and the pharmaceutical forms (if applicable), their intended use and maximum quantities to be possessed at any one time, the training and experience of the individual users, the radiation-detection instruments available, and the personnel monitoring procedures. In addition, a description of the laboratory facilities, the handling of equipment, and the waste-disposal procedures, as well as the radiation-protection program, is required.

If radioactive material is to be administered to humans, a specific license issued only to physicians is required. Title 10, Part 35.14 of the CFR states that an application for a specific license for diagnostic use of by-product material for uptake, dilution, excretion, or scanning procedures will be considered as an application for all of the diagnostic uses listed in 35.100 if the applicant meets the requirements of proper training and experience, demonstrates availability of appropriate equipment for performance of the procedures, and has appropriate monitoring equipment, waste-disposal procedures, radiation-protection program, and access to hospital facilities. The NRC in agreement with the Food and Drug Administration (FDA) regulates which radionuclides and pharmaceutical forms are listed in 35.100. If a physician wishes to use either a radionuclide or a pharmaceutical not so listed, he must apply individually for each item.

An individual who plans to work with radionuclides at any institution such as a hospital must apply for an NRC (or other agency, such as city or state) license through that institution. Clinical programs sponsored by medical institutions are subject to a review by a radioactive materials committee, which must approve the license application. It is still true that a license is issued to an individual and must be specifically obtained for each radionuclide and for each pharmaceutical form not named in 35.100. However, physicians in training may participate in an institutional program. The institution, however, is responsible for the individual's compliance with provisions of the license.

Institutions that meet the requirements regarding staffing and facilities may obtain a license of broad scope. This license enables them to establish a radioactive materials committee, which may authorize specific members of their staff to work with radionuclides without special application to the regulatory agency for each individual user. Broad licenses can be issued for work involving animals only or for animal work and human use both.

A distinction is made regarding the use of radioactive materials in a live person, in vivo, and the use of such materials in laboratory tests involving tissues or fluids extracted from a living person, in vitro. Licenses may be issued to use certain radionuclides, such as ^{125}I, in vitro, but not in vivo. Part 35 of Title 10 governs only in vivo uses.

Any institution that uses radionuclides must have a radiation-safety program conducted under the authority of a radioisotopes committee and implemented by a radiation protection officer (RPO). The duties of the RPO reach into every aspect of radiation safety. To name but a few, the RPO prepares regulations, advises on matters of radiation protection, maintains a system of accountability for all radioactive material from procurement to disposal, inspects work spaces and handling procedures, determines personnel radiation exposures, monitors environmental radiation levels, and institutes corrective action in the event of accidents or emergencies. Since all users of radionuclides are subject to periodic inspections and committee reviews, the RPO's duties are of the utmost importance.

Certain general not broad licenses are issued to any physician for specific diagnostic uses of specially prepared radiopharmaceuticals in prepackaged individual doses. Examples of this are ^{131}I as sodium iodide for measurement of thyroid uptake, or as iodinated human serum albumin (I-HSA) for determination of blood and blood-plasma volume. The physician must fill out a registration form stating that he has and is competent to operate appropriate radiation measuring instruments. His authorization is valid only when he has received a properly stamped copy of his registration form from the NRC. At no time does the general license authorize a physician to administer radiopharmaceuticals to a woman confirmed pregnant or to a person under 18 years of age. The maximum levels of activity that the physician may possess at any one time are limited to 7.4 MBq of ^{131}I, ^{125}I, and chromium-51 (^{51}Cr) and to 0.2 MBq of cobalt-58 (^{58}Co) and ^{60}Co. These general license holders are also exempt from the radiation-protection standards directed to other licensees. Last, general licenses are also issued by the NRC for use of ^{131}I or ^{125}I for in vitro clinical or laboratory testing.

RECORD KEEPING

Once a person—usually a physician—has received authorization to use radionuclides, he becomes directly responsible for compliance with all the regulations governing the safe use of the radionuclides in his possession. He is also responsible for the safe use of those radionuclides by others who, under his supervision, work with the material.

A complete record must be kept on each radionuclide from its receipt through its final disposition. For this reason, in a large institution such as a hospital, the ordering and receiving of radionuclides are usually done through some centralized system overseen by the RPO. Each licensee then receives his radionuclides from the central receiving area. Each authorized user must then keep a complete record of how the radionuclide is used. Patient doses must be carefully noted together with the pharmaceutical form in which they are administered. A separate master record is kept for each radionuclide. In this record, amount received, amount used for particular purposes and that purpose—e.g., as patient dose, for use with animals, for laboratory work—and amount disposed of are carefully noted. At all times, an inventory of amount of radioactive material on hand must be kept, and this inventory must be ready to be submitted to inspectors upon request.

When a generator system is used for obtaining a radionuclide, records must also be kept of the chemical and radioactive purity of the eluate (the generator product). For example, in the molybdenum-technetium (^{99}Mo-^{99m}Tc) generator system, it is necessary to check for and to record the purity of the product, ^{99m}Tc. Since the eluate should contain no ^{99}Mo, this procedure is usually known as checking for molybdenum breakthrough. In addition, this generator contains an alumina column. Since alumina is nonradioactive, its breakthrough must be tested for by chemical means. Alumina breakthrough is rare and is not usually tested for on a routine basis in this type of generator system.

Equally important, records must be kept of personnel exposure, radiation surveys or wipe tests, instrument calibration, waste disposal, and radiation incidents. In an institutional setting these records are usually maintained or at least overseen by the RPO. The records kept with respect to all radiation activities represent the main proof that an authorized user has of his compliance with the radiation-protection regulations. They are, consequently, important for legal purposes as well as for effective administration of the radiation-protection program.

AREA POSTING AND RADIONUCLIDE LABELLING

The law requires that certain types of signs be used to warn of danger or of possible danger from the presence of radiation. The requirements include all areas where radiation in any form may be encountered and is not restricted only to areas where radionuclides are used. Warning signs are necessary because individuals might otherwise be unaware of the presence of radiation. At the same time, the sign used should reflect the actual radiation danger present and should not be more or less serious than

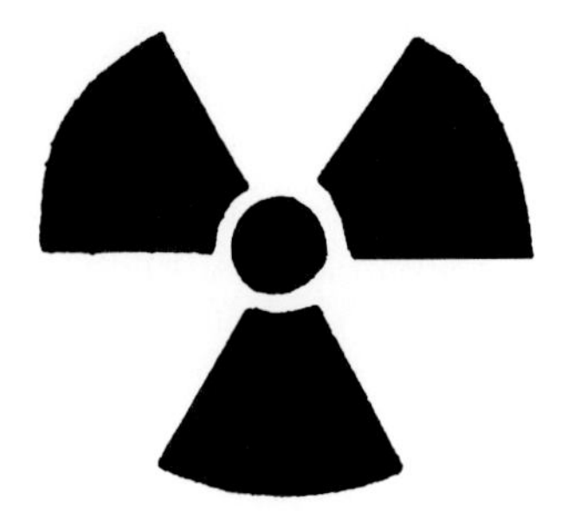

Figure 9.1: The three-bladed radioactive caution symbol.

needed. All signs must bear the three-bladed trefoil symbol of the exploding atom, which is the radioactive caution symbol. This symbol is usually colored magenta or purple on a yellow background (Fig. 9.1).

The types of signs and labels used are as follows:

1. *Restricted Area*: This type of sign may be used but is *not required*. It is appropriate when a person might receive radiation in excess of 20 μSv per hour if he were continually present in the area, but not in excess of 50 μSv per hour. The area itself must be controlled by license.
2. *Caution: Radiation Area:* This sign is used but again *not required* when the personnel having access to the area may receive in any 1 hour a dose of 50 μSv or in any 5 consecutive days a dose in excess of 1.0 mSv to the major portion of the body. The area itself must be controlled by a license. It is useful to post Unauthorized Persons Prohibited signs at the entrance to such areas.
3. *High Radiation Area*: This sign is required if a person in the area could receive a dose to a major portion of the body in excess of 1.0 mSv in any 1 hour. Such areas also require audible or visible alarm signals, such as warning tones or flashing, colored lights.
4. *Caution: Radioactive Material* (room): In general, rooms in which radioactive materials are used and/or stored must be posted

with this sign in addition to any others that may also be required. However, small quantities are exempted but these exemptions are usually not applicable in medical work.

5. *Airborne Radioactivity Area*: This sign is required if airborne radioactivity exceeds at any time the maximum permissible concentrations listed in Table 8.1 for 40 hours of occupational exposure. It is also required if the average over the number of hours in any week during which individuals are in the area exceeds 25% of the maximum permissible concentration.
6. *Caution: Radioactive Material* (label): This label is required on any container in which quantities of radionuclide are transported, stored, or used. Even refrigerators and containers for waste disposal should be so labelled. When the containers are used for storage, the labels should state, additionally, the nuclide(s) present, the amount of activity of each nuclide, and the date of each assay.

STORAGE AND DELIVERY

Ideally, radionuclides should be delivered to a central location where contents of the package are inspected, monitored, logged, and stored by trained personnel until the material is picked up by the authorized user. Upon receipt, all containers of radionuclides should be carefully checked for evidence of leakage or breakage.

Should delivery be made to the general receiving area of an institution, the package should be logged in and quickly transferred to the user or to a controlled storage area until it is delivered to or picked up by the licensee. Clearly visible signs giving specific instructions pertaining to the handling of radioactive material packages should be posted conspicuously in the receiving area. Records should also be kept of the names of the person receiving the package and the person to whom it is transferred or who places it in a locked storage area.

When radionuclides requiring a Radioactive Materials label are to be stored, the areas chosen must be locked and protected against fire, explosion, or flooding. Radionuclides must also be stored in adequately shielded containers. The practical rule is to shield stored materials so the radiation level is less than 50 μSv per hour at a distance of 1 foot from the shield's surface. It is most desirable to keep the radiation exposure level below 1.0 mSv per hour; otherwise, the storage area must be treated as a high-radiation area. The RPO must be informed of any transfer of radionuclides to a new area, i.e., previously undesignated areas, for storage.

Whenever radionuclides are ordered, a copy of the user's license must be kept on file by the vendor. It is the vendor's responsibility to see that only those radionuclides covered by the user's license are delivered.

TRANSPORT

Government regulations pertaining to packaging and transporting of radionuclides are myriad and confusing. The packaging regulations are contained in Title 10 Part 71 of the CFR and are administered by the NRC. The transporting regulations are contained in Title 49 Parts 100–199 of the CFR and are administered by the U.S. Department of Transportation. In addition, agreement states and, in the case of New York City, agreement cities have added further regulations to those already in existence. Thus packaging and transporting of radionuclides are fraught with all manner of considerations. In addition, Title 10 Part 36 regulates the export and import of byproduct material.

It is possible, under stringent circumstances, to send radionuclides through the U.S. Postal Service. A brief summary of the mailing regulations is contained in the U.S. Postal Service pamphlet, Radioactive Matter, Publication 6, April, 1971. It is more usual to send radionuclides via a carrier licensed specially for carrying them. If the cargo-carrying vehicle is not used exclusively for transporting radionuclides, the dose rate must be less than 2.0 mSv per hour at surface of the package and 0.1 mSv per hour at 3 feet from the package. If, however, the transporting is done by a vehicle used exclusively for this purpose and is loaded and unloaded by properly trained personnel, the dose rate can be as high as 10 mSv per hour at 3 feet from surface of the package, 2.0 mSv per hour at any point on the external surface of the vehicle, 0.10 mSv per hour at 6 feet from the external surface of the vehicle, and 0.02 mSv per hour in any normally occupied position in the vehicle.

Licensed users who send radionuclides by taxi or other vehicles that primarily carry passengers must check that the carrier has the appropriate commercial license for transporting radioactive materials. Proper shipping papers and other record-keeping requirements should also be observed. If a user is licensed to use his own car for transporting radionuclides, his insurance policy should be checked for possible exclusion clauses with regard to accidents involving radioactive materials.

If radionuclides are carried on foot from one institution to another, proper precautions, such as the use of shatterproof containers and adequate shielding, must be observed. The dose rate at 3 feet from the container must be less than 0.1 mSv per hour, and tests must be made to determine that no removable contamination exists on the surface of the container. When such material is transported by foot messenger, it should be routed to encounter the minimum number of pedestrians.

Packages containing radionuclides in amounts that are not mailable must be labelled according to the following method. The labels are diamond-shaped and bear radioactive caution signs. In all, three different labels must appear: (1) radioactive white I; this label is all white with one red stripe in the lower half of the diamond. It is used on packages where the dose rate at any point on the external surface is less than 5 μSv per hour; (2) radioactive yellow II; here the upper half of the label is yellow; the lower is white and contains two red stripes. This

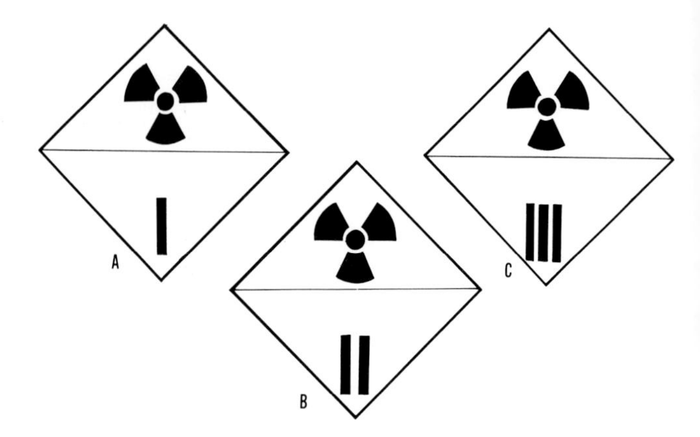

Figure 9.2: Radioactive caution labels for the transport of radionuclides. A. Radioactive White I: the label is all white with a black three-bladed radioactive caution symbol in the upper half and one red stripe in the lower half. B. Radioactive Yellow II: the upper half is yellow with a black three-bladed radioactive caution symbol in the upper half; the lower half is white with two red stripes. C. Radioactive Yellow III: the upper half is yellow with a black three-bladed radioactive caution symbol in the upper half; the lower half is white with three red stripes.

label is used on packages where the dose rate is between 5 and 100 μSv per hour on the surface and less than 5 μSv per hour at 3 feet; (3) the radioactive yellow III; this label is yellow on the upper half of the diamond and white below. It contains three red stripes in the white half. This label signifies that the dose rate at the surface of the package is greater than 100 μSv per hour or that the dose rate is greater than 5 μSv per hour at 3 feet. The dose rate, however, cannot exceed 500 μSv per hour at 3 feet. Vehicles transporting packages with radioactive yellow III labels must display radioactive signs. Figure 9.2 shows the three types of labels. Additionally, each radionuclide is given a transport group designation, and each aggregate shipment is given a fissile class.

These concepts are defined in Title 10 Part 71 of the CFR.

RADIONUCLIDES AND ANIMALS

When animals are injected with radionuclides, contamination-control procedures should always be employed. One common method is to use trays lined with absorbent material. The cages of such animals must have labels stating the radionuclide, quantity of material injected per animal, date of injection, and name of the licensed user. Special cages, such as metabolic-type cages, should be used any time contamination is a problem. The radioactive animals should be housed separately from other animals.

It is important that adequate ventilation be provided when radioactive substance in animals kept after injection may become volatile and hence dispersed into the area housing them. Animal handlers should be instructed by the authorized investigator with respect to dose levels, time limitations in the area, and handling requirements of animal carcasses and excreta.

If the animal excreta are not mixed with sawdust or wood-shavings and are below the limits given in Table 8.1, they may be disposed of in the sewage system. Otherwise, they should be placed in plastic bags and disposed of as solid waste. The animal carcasses should be dealt with as solid waste.

WASTE DISPOSAL

In the radiologic and health sciences, the radioactive waste material generated usually has a very low level of radioactivity. In other words, the wastes have so little radioactivity left that they may be disposed of directly by release to the air, by disposal through sewage systems, or by burial in the ground.

Disposal of liquid wastes into the sanitary sewage system or dispersal of gaseous wastes into the atmosphere is permissible as long as the concentration of radioactivity is less than that considered safe for an adult to drink or to breathe. A summary of the maximum permissible concentrations for some radionuclides in air and water is given in Table 8.1. In the case of liquids, allowance can be made for other sewage discharged in the same building if that sewage dilutes radioactive waste. In other words the total daily amount of sewage from the facility must be known as well as the total amount of radioactive waste discharged by the entire facility. Solutions or gaseous wastes which, because of their high radiation level, cannot be released at once can be allowed to decay until the radiation level is below the acceptable maximum. The usual rule of thumb is to wait 10 half-lives. This method requires a shielded storage space. Liquids or gaseous wastes not disposed of in the preceding manner must be solidified for disposal with the solid waste material.

As regards solid waste materials, general practice is to package and transport them to designated burial sites. It is also common practice first to decay these solid wastes in properly shielded areas within each laboratory for 10 half-lives, as noted previously. Afterward, solid wastes, including test tubes, are taken to a location designated for the entire complex, from which site they are taken for burial on a regular basis. The complex either has a burial site and procedures strictly regulated by law in the form of a license, or hires an outside concern licensed to dispose of the waste.

If an outside vendor is employed, he is responsible for collection from the central site and disposal of the radioactive waste material. In this case, the vendor is strictly regulated by law and is responsible for safe burial of the refuse. However, nothing should be placed for disposal until it has decayed for approximately 10 half-lives.

BIBLIOGRAPHY

Code of Federal Regulations, Titles 10 and 49.

Shapiro, J.: Practical aspects of the use of radionuclides (Part V). In Radiation Protection. Cambridge, MA, Harvard University Press, 1972.

chapter 10

INTERNAL DOSIMETRY

Radionuclides are generally administered internally for diagnostic or therapeutic reasons. At the same time, radiation workers may unintentionally acquire radionuclides internally. In either case, it is important to calculate the radiation dose received not only by the total body but also by individual organs. In order to accomplish this goal, the Society of Nuclear Medicine has established the Medical Internal Radiation Dose (MIRD) Committee and charged this committee with developing standard methods for this calculation. This committee's results are published in pamphlets issued as supplements to the *Journal of Nuclear Medicine*. The method detailed here for calculating absorbed dose from internal radionuclides uses the latest work of the MIRD Committee.*

EFFECTIVE HALF-LIFE

In Chapter 1 radioactivity was defined as the rate of decay of a radionuclide. This decay rate may be expressed in the following manner:

$$A = A_0 e^{-\lambda t} \tag{10.1}$$

*Pamphlet No. 11, issued October, 1975, contains absorbed dose tables for many different radionuclides. Two of those tables, for ^{99m}Tc and for ^{123}I, are reprinted here. In the event that a particular absorbed dose calculation cannot be performed using the tables of Pamphlet No. 11, the earlier pamphlets—Nos. 4, 5, 6, and 10—should be used.

where A is activity at time t, A_0 is initial activity, λ is probability for a particular radionuclide to decay, and t is time. λ is a constant, known as the decay constant, which is specific to each particular radionuclide. The resemblance between this equation and equation 7.7 is to be noted: the form is the same; only the names of the physical quantities have been changed. Thus, this equation can follow all the same mathematical manipulation done following or with equation 7.7.

In Chapter 7 a half-value layer, or thickness t/2, was defined. The HVL was the thickness of material that reduced the number N_0 of photons to one-half of its original value. A similar quantity can be defined here. Since the rate of radioactive decay is directly proportional to the number of nuclei of the particular radionuclide present, the activity of the radionuclide decreases as time passes and more nuclei have decayed. When one-half of the nuclei in the sample have decayed, the rate of decay is also equal to one-half of its original value. The time for half of the nuclei to decay is known as the half-life of that particular radionuclide.

Symbolically,

$$A = \frac{A_0}{2} \text{ at } t = t_{1/2} \qquad (10.2)$$

and from equation 10.1

$$\frac{A_0}{2} = A_0 e^{-\lambda t_{1/2}} \qquad (10.3)$$

Cancelling A_0, we obtain

$$1/2 = e^{-\lambda t_{1/2}} \qquad (10.4)$$

Taking the natural logarithm of both sides, we have

$$\ln 1/2 = \ln 1 - \ln 2 = -\ln 2 = -\lambda t_{1/2} \qquad (10.5)$$

and, as before equation 7.10

$$\frac{\ln 2}{\lambda} = t_{1/2} \qquad (10.6)$$

This $t_{1/2}$ is known as the physical half-life, $t_{1/2p}$, of the radionuclide because it is a property of the radionuclide itself.

When radionuclides are used in a biologic system, they can be eliminated from that system by metabolic processes as well as decay. For each radiopharmaceutical form, a metabolic rate can be defined using the same parameters as those in the preceding equations—namely, a biologic decay constant λ_b and a biologic half-life $t_{1/2b}$. Unfortunately, nature is not always kind and sometimes the biologic activity cannot be expressed in terms of one simple exponential, as in equation 10.1. However, it can be expressed as some linear sum of exponentials. For simplicity, in this discussion it has been assumed that the metabolic rates can be fully described by one value of λ_b and one $t_{1/2b}$. In general, the error made by this assumption is not large.

In order then to describe the life of a radionuclide in a living system, the physical half-life must be combined with the biologic half-life. In terms of the decay constants this combining is easy:

$$\lambda_{eff} = \lambda_b + \lambda_p \qquad (10.7)$$

where $\lambda_{effective}$ is the total probability that a particular radionuclide will be eliminated, either through metabolic processes, quantized by $\lambda_{biologic}$ or through radioactive decay, quantized by $\lambda_{physical}$. Since the half-lives are related to the decay constants through equation 10.6, an expression for the effective half-life, $t_{1/2eff}$, can be obtained. It is

$$t_{1/2eff} = \frac{t_{1/2p} \cdot t_{1/2b}}{t_{1/2p} + t_{1/2b}} \qquad (10.8)$$

One attractive feature of this expression is: If one half-life is much larger than the other, $t_{1/2eff}$ is equal to the other half-life. For example, suppose in a certain situation, $t_{1/2b}$ is much larger than $t_{1/2p}$. Then

$$t_{1/2p} + t_{1/2b} \cong t_{1/2b} \tag{10.9}$$

So equation 10.8 gives, using equation 10.9

$$t_{1/2eff} \cong \frac{t_{1/2p} \cdot t_{1/2b}}{t_{1/2b}} \tag{10.10}$$

and hence, cancelling $t_{1/2b}$ in both numerator and denominator,

$$t_{1/2eff} \cong t_{1/2p} \tag{10.11}$$

When calculating internal dose, $t_{1/2eff}$ must be used. Therefore, it is necessary to know or to approximate the value of $t_{1/2b}$, which requires a knowledge of the physiology of the living system in question. Once $t_{1/2b}$ is decided, then $t_{1/2eff}$ can be calculated from equation 10.8.

STANDARD MAN

Internal-dose calculations are based on a geometric rendering of the human body and its organs. When a radionuclide in some pharmaceutical form is introduced into the body, it distributes itself either throughout the entire body or throughout an entire organ or organs. For this reason, the radioactive source cannot be considered as a point source. In order, therefore, to simplify the calculation, the MIRD Committee has adopted from the International Commission on Radiological Protection (ICRP) a geometrically symmetric version of the human body and of human organs based on the norm that standard man weighs 70 kilograms. Figure 10.1 shows standard man. Table 10.1 gives organ masses assigned to standard man; dose calculations are available for only these organs.

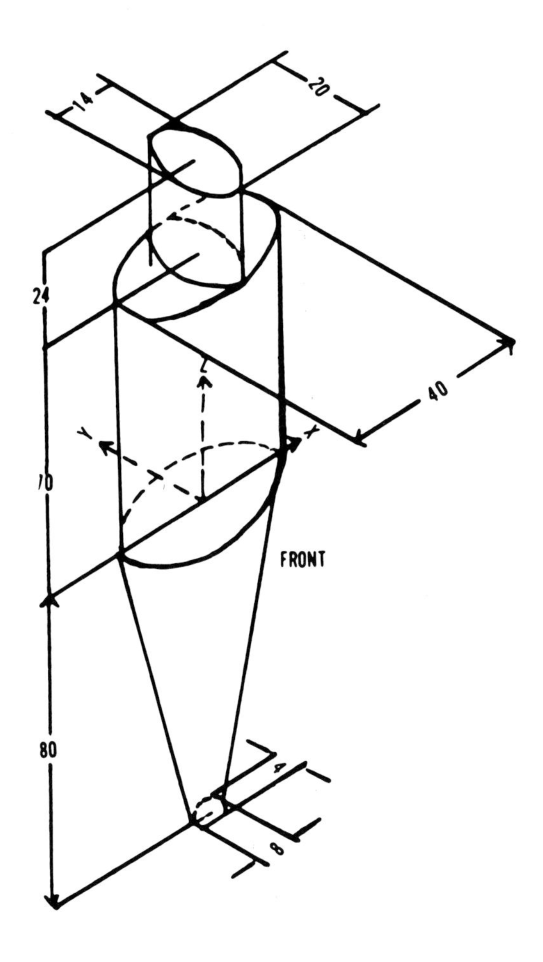

Figure 10.1: The Adult Human Phantom (dimensions in centimeters). (From MIRD Pamphlet No. 5, 1969. Reproduced with permission of the Society of Nuclear Medicine.)

Table 10.1

Masses of Body Organs Used in the Reference Man Report

Body Organs	*Organ Mass (kg)*
Adrenals	0.014
Bladder	
Wall	0.045
Contents	0.200
Gastrointestinal tract	
Stomach	
Wall	0.150
Contents	0.250
Small intestine and contents	
Wall	0.640
Contents	0.400
Upper large intestine	
Wall	0.210
Contents	0.220
Lower large intestine	
Wall	0.160
Contents	0.135
Kidneys (both)	0.310
Liver	1.800
Lungs (both, including blood)	1.000
Other tissue	48.000
Ovaries (both)	0.011
Pancreas	0.100
Salivary glands	0.085
Skeleton	10.000
Cortical bone	4.000
Trabecular bone	1.000
Red marrow	1.500
Yellow marrow	1.500
Cartilage	1.100
Other constituents	0.900
Spleen	0.180
Testes	0.035
Thyroid	0.020
Uterus	0.080
Total body	70.000

From MIRD Pamphlet No. 11, 1975. Reproduced with permission of the Society of Nuclear Medicine.

CUMULATED ACTIVITY

The dose that is absorbed internally is dependent upon a number of factors. Chief among these factors is activity administered to the patient and half-life of the nuclide. The type of radiation emitted, as well as its geometric distribution, is accounted for in another part of the calculation.

When activity is administered to a patient, it diminishes in time both because of physical decay of the radionuclide and because of metabolic processes occurring in the person. From equation 10.1 the activity at any time can be expressed as

$$A = A_o e^{-\lambda t} \quad (10.1)$$

If $\lambda_{effective}$ is now used to express the decrease from initial activity A_o to activity at any time A as a result of both physical and metabolic decay, one obtains

$$A = A_o e^{-\lambda_{eff} t} \quad (10.12)$$

To find the activity at every time from some initial time $t_1 = 0$ to some future time t_2, equation 10.12 must be integrated with respect to time. Thus

$$A \text{ (cumulated over time)} = \int_{t_1 = 0}^{t_2} A_o e^{-\lambda_{eff} t} dt \quad (10.13)$$

If t_2 is now taken to be very long with respect to $t_{\frac{1}{2}eff}$, then t_2 is approximately equal to infinity and

$$A_{cum} = \frac{A_o}{\lambda_{eff}} \quad (10.14)$$

This expression is used in the internal-dose calculation. In the same manner that equation 10.6 was derived, it is found that

$$\frac{\ln 2}{\lambda_{eff}} = t_{\frac{1}{2}eff} \quad (10.15)$$

and, rearranging the preceding equation

$$\frac{1}{\lambda_{eff}} = \frac{t_{½eff}}{\ln 2} = 1.44\ t_{½eff} \qquad (10.16)$$

Hence,

$$A_{cum} = A_o\ 1.44 t_{½eff} \qquad (10.17)$$

or alternatively, using equation 10.8

$$A_{cum} = A_o\ 1.44\ \frac{t_{½b} \cdot t_{½p}}{t_{½b} + t_{½p}} \qquad (10.18)$$

In determining the absorbed dose from internal radioactivity, equation 10.17 is used.

"S": THE ABSORBED DOSE PER UNIT CUMULATED ACTIVITY

The value of absorbed dose per unit cumulated activity is the quantity that has been calculated and tabulated by the MIRD Committee. In order to make the calculation feasible, certain assumptions have been made.*

The "S" tables presented in Pamphlet No. 11, however, are accurate enough for determining dose to a particular organ or to the total body in most practical situations. At present, the MIRD calculations are done only for larger organs of the body and the total body and for certain selected radionuclides. However, the organs selected are of the most interest, and the radionuclides selected are the ones most commonly used.

The high penetrating ability of photons makes untenable the assumption that they deposit their energy in the organ in which they are emitted. Consequently, geometric and statistical assumptions play a large part in determining where, within the

*If more accuracy is required than is provided by the present set of tables, other calculation methods, such as the one presented in MIRD Pamphlet No. 5, must be used.

body, photons deposit their energy, if at all.* For calculating absorbed dose due to photons, the MIRD Committee has used a standard statistical calculation method known as the Monte Carlo technique.† A detailed knowledge of the assumptions made is not necessary for correct use of the tables.

For electrons, the MIRD Committee has assumed that all their energy is deposited within the organ in which they are emitted. This assumption is valid except in the case of organs with contents and walls, e.g., the large and small intestines, and in the case of bones and bone marrow. In these instances, the committee has made special assumptions.‡

Finally, the absorbed-dose tables are based on the assumption that radionuclides are distributed uniformly within the organ or organs in question or throughout the total body. The implications of this and other assumptions are described in MIRD Pamphlet No. 11. However, the S values given in the tables of MIRD Pamphlet No. 11 are quite sufficient for ordinary calculation of patient and radiation-worker doses.

USE OF THE MIRD TABLES

To calculate absorbed dose from an internally administered radionuclide, the following formula is used:

$$D_{\text{absorbed dose}} = A_{\text{cum}}(\text{cumulated activity}) \cdot S\ (\text{absorbed dose per cumulated activity}) \qquad (10.19)$$

Using equation 10.17, one obtains

$$D = A_0\ 1.44\ t_{½\text{eff}} S$$

*The geometric assumptions made by the MIRD Committee are embodied in their estimate of standard man and are explicitly given in MIRD Pamphlet No. 5.

†The particular Monte Carlo estimates made are described in MIRD Pamphlet No. 11.

‡These assumptions are specified in MIRD Pamphlet No. 11, but again detailed knowledge of them is not necessary.

Table 10.2

S, Absorbed Dose per Unit Cumulated Activity, (Rad/μCi-hr)
Technetium-99m Half-Life 6.03 Hours

	Source Organs									
			Intestinal Tract							
Target Organs	*Adrenals*	*Bladder Contents*	*Stomach Contents*	*SI Contents*	*ULI Contents*	*LLI Contents*	*Kidneys*	*Liver*	*Lungs*	*Other Tissue (Muscle)*
Adrenals	3.1E-03	1.5E-07	2.7E-06	1.0E-06	9.1E-07	3.6E-07	1.1E-05	4.5E-06	2.7E-06	1.4E-06
Bladder wall	1.3E-07	1.6E-04	2.7E-07	2.6E-06	2.2E-06	6.9E-06	2.8E-07	1.6E-07	3.6E-08	1.8E-06
Bone (total)	2.0E-06	9.2E-07	9.0E-07	1.3E-06	1.1E-06	1.6E-06	1.4E-06	1.1E-06	1.5E-06	9.8E-07
GI (stomach wall)	2.9E-06	2.7E-07	1.3E-04	3.7E-06	3.8E-06	1.8E-06	3.6E-06	1.9E-06	1.8E-06	1.3E-06
GI (SI)	8.3E-07	3.0E-06	2.7E-06	7.8E-05	1.7E-05	9.4E-06	2.9E-06	1.6E-06	1.9E-07	1.5E-06
GI (ULI wall)	9.3E-07	2.2E-06	3.5E-06	2.4E-05	1.3E-04	4.2E-06	2.9E-06	2.5E-06	2.2E-07	1.6E-06
GI (LLI wall)	2.2E-07	7.4E-06	1.2E-06	7.3E-06	3.2E-06	1.9E-04	7.2E-07	2.3E-07	7.1E-08	1.7E-06
Kidneys	1.1E-05	2.6E-07	3.5E-06	3.2E-06	2.8E-06	8.6E-07	1.9E-04	3.9E-06	8.4E-07	1.3E-06
Liver	4.9E-06	1.7E-07	2.0E-06	1.8E-06	2.6E-06	2.5E-07	3.9E-06	4.6E-05	2.5E-06	1.1E-06
Lungs	2.4E-06	2.4E-08	1.7E-06	2.2E-07	2.6E-07	7.9E-08	8.5E-07	2.5E-06	5.2E-05	1.3E-06
Marrow (red)	3.6E-06	2.2E-06	1.6E-06	4.3E-06	3.7E-06	5.1E-06	3.8E-06	1.6E-06	1.9E-06	2.0E-06
Other tissues (muscles)	1.4E-06	1.8E-06	1.4E-06	1.5E-06	1.5E-06	1.7E-06	1.3E-06	1.1E-06	1.3E-06	2.7E-06
Ovaries	6.1E-07	7.3E-06	5.0E-07	1.1E-05	1.2E-05	1.8E-05	1.1E-06	4.5E-07	9.4E-08	2.0E-06
Pancreas	9.0E-06	2.3E-07	1.8E-05	2.1E-06	2.3E-06	7.4E-07	6.6E-06	4.2E-06	2.6E-06	1.8E-06
Skin	5.1E-07	5.5E-07	4.4E-07	4.1E-07	4.1E-07	4.8E-07	5.3E-07	4.9E-07	5.3E-07	7.2E-07
Spleen	6.3E-06	6.6E-07	1.0E-05	1.5E-06	1.4E-06	8.0E-07	8.6E-06	9.2E-07	2.3E-06	1.4E-06
Testes	3.2E-08	4.7E-06	5.1E-08	3.1E-07	2.7E-07	1.8E-06	8.8E-08	6.2E-08	7.9E-09	1.1E-06
Thyroid	1.3E-07	2.1E-09	8.7E-08	1.5E-08	1.6E-08	5.4E-09	4.8E-08	1.5E-07	9.2E-07	1.3E-06
Uterus (nongravid)	1.1E-06	1.6E-05	7.7E-07	9.6E-06	5.4E-06	7.1E-06	9.4E-07	3.9E-07	8.2E-08	2.3E-06
Total body	2.2E-06	1.9E-06	1.9E-06	2.4E-06	2.2E-06	2.3E-06	2.2E-06	2.2E-06	2.0E-06	1.9E-06

Target Organs	Source Organs									
			Skeleton							
	Ovaries	*Pancreas*	*Red Marrow*	*Cortical Bone*	*Trabecular Bone*	*Skin*	*Spleen*	*Testes*	*Thyroid*	*Total Body*
Adrenals	3.3E-07	9.1E-06	2.3E-06	1.1E-06	1.1E-06	6.8E-07	6.3E-06	3.2E-08	1.3E-07	2.3E-06
Bladder wall	7.2E-06	1.4E-07	9.9E-07	5.1E-07	5.1E-07	4.9E-07	1.2E-07	4.8E-06	2.1E-09	2.3E-06
Bone (total)	1.5E-06	1.5E-06	4.0E-06	1.2E-05	1.0E-05	9.9E-07	1.1E-06	9.2E-07	1.0E-06	2.5E-06
GI (stomach wall)	8.1E-07	1.8E-05	9.5E-07	5.5E-07	5.5E-07	5.4E-07	1.0E-05	3.2E-08	4.5E-08	2.2E-06
GI (SI)	1.2E-05	1.8E-06	2.6E-06	7.3E-07	7.3E-07	4.5E-07	1.4E-06	3.6E-07	9.3E-09	2.5E-06
GI (ULI wall)	1.1E-05	2.1E-06	2.1E-06	6.9E-07	6.9E-07	4.6E-07	1.4E-06	3.1E-07	1.1E-08	2.4E-06
GI (LLI wall)	1.5E-05	5.7E-07	2.9E-06	1.0E-06	1.0E-06	4.8E-07	6.1E-07	2.7E-06	4.3E-09	2.3E-06
Kidneys	9.2E-07	6.6E-06	2.2E-06	8.2E-07	8.2E-07	5.7E-07	9.1E-06	4.0E-08	3.4E-08	2.2E-06
Liver	5.4E-07	4.4E-06	9.2E-07	6.6E-07	6.6E-07	5.3E-07	9.8E-07	3.1E-08	9.3E-08	2.2E-06
Lungs	6.0E-08	2.5E-06	1.2E-06	9.4E-07	9.4E-07	5.8E-07	2.3E-06	6.6E-09	9.4E-07	2.0E-06
Marrow (red)	5.5E-06	2.8E-06	3.1E-05	4.1E-06	9.1E-06	9.5E-07	1.7E-06	7.3E-07	1.1E-06	2.9E-06
Other tissues (muscles)	2.0E-06	1.8E-06	1.2E-06	9.8E-07	9.8E-07	7.2E-07	1.4E-06	1.1E-06	1.3E-06	1.9E-06
Ovaries	4.2E-03	4.1E-07	3.2E-06	7.1E-07	7.1E-07	3.8E-07	4.0E-07	0.0	4.9E-09	2.4E-06
Pancreas	5.0E-07	5.8E-04	1.7E-06	8.5E-07	8.5E-07	4.4E-07	1.9E-05	5.5E-08	7.2E-08	2.4E-06
Skin	4.1E-07	4.0E-07	5.9E-07	6.5E-07	6.5E-07	1.6E-05	4.7E-07	1.4E-06	7.3E-07	1.3E-06
Spleen	4.9E-07	1.9E-05	9.2E-07	5.8E-07	5.8E-07	5.4E-07	3.3E-04	1.7E-08	1.1E-07	2.2E-06
Testes	0.0	5.5E-08	4.5E-07	6.4E-07	6.4E-07	9.1E-07	4.8E-08	1.4E-03	5.0E-10	1.7E-06
Thyroid	4.9E-09	1.2E-07	6.8E-07	7.9E-07	7.9E-07	6.9E-07	8.7E-08	5.0E-10	2.3E-03	1.5E-06
Uterus (nongravid)	2.1E-05	5.3E-07	2.2E-06	5.7E-07	5.7E-07	4.0E-07	4.0E-07	0.0	4.6E-09	2.6E-06
Total body	2.6E-06	2.6E-06	2.2E-06	2.0E-06	2.0E-06	1.3E-06	2.2E-06	1.9E-06	1.8E-06	2.0E-06

Decay data revised—March, 1972. Reference—MIRD Pamphlet No. 10.

Date of issue, 05-13-75. Reproduced with permission of the Society of Nuclear Medicine (MIRD No. 11).

Table 10.3

S, Absorbed Dose per Unit Cumulated Activity, (Rad/μCi-hr)
Iodine-123 Half-Life 13.0 Hours

	Source Organs									
			Intestinal Tract							
Target Organs	*Adrenals*	*Bladder Contents*	*Stomach Contents*	*SI Contents*	*ULI Contents*	*LLI Contents*	*Kidneys*	*Liver*	*Lungs*	*Other Tissue (Muscle)*
Adrenals	5.3E-03	2.0E-07	3.1E-06	1.4E-06	1.1E-06	4.5E-07	1.7E-05	6.6E-06	3.3E-06	2.2E-06
Bladder wall	1.5E-07	2.8E-04	3.1E-07	3.3E-06	2.6E-06	8.3E-06	3.4E-07	1.9E-07	4.9E-08	2.5E-06
Bone (total)	2.7E-06	1.0E-06	1.1E-06	1.5E-06	1.4E-06	2.3E-06	1.8E-06	1.4E-06	2.0E-06	1.3E-06
GI (stomach wall)	3.6E-06	3.2E-07	2.2E-04	4.8E-06	5.3E-06	2.2E-06	4.3E-06	2.3E-06	2.5E-06	1.8E-06
GI (SI)	9.8E-07	3.6E-06	3.3E-06	1.3E-04	2.6E-05	1.4E-05	3.6E-06	2.0E-06	2.3E-07	2.1E-06
GI (ULI wall)	1.1E-06	2.7E-06	4.7E-06	4.1E-05	2.2E-04	6.3E-06	3.5E-06	3.2E-06	2.8E-07	2.2E-06
GI (LLI wall)	2.6E-07	9.8E-06	1.5E-06	1.1E-05	4.4E-06	3.2E-04	9.0E-07	2.7E-07	9.6E-08	2.3E-06
Kidneys	1.7E-05	3.2E-07	4.3E-06	3.9E-06	3.5E-06	1.1E-06	3.4E-04	5.1E-06	1.0E-06	2.0E-06
Liver	6.8E-06	2.2E-07	2.5E-06	2.3E-06	3.3E-06	3.1E-07	5.1E-06	7.9E-05	3.4E-06	1.5E-06
Lungs	3.2E-06	3.0E-08	2.3E-06	2.7E-07	3.1E-07	9.5E-08	1.0E-06	3.6E-06	9.2E-05	2.0E-06
Marrow (red)	4.8E-06	2.5E-06	1.9E-06	5.3E-06	4.6E-06	7.6E-06	4.8E-06	2.0E-06	2.5E-06	2.8E-06
Other tissues (muscles)	2.2E-06	2.5E-06	1.9E-06	2.1E-06	2.0E-06	2.3E-06	2.0E-06	1.5E-06	2.0E-06	4.4E-06
Ovaries	6.9E-07	9.5E-06	5.7E-07	1.5E-05	1.7E-05	3.0E-05	1.3E-06	5.2E-07	1.2E-07	2.9E-06
Pancreas	1.2E-05	2.9E-07	2.7E-05	2.4E-06	2.8E-06	8.6E-07	8.5E-06	5.4E-06	3.3E-06	2.6E-06
Skin	7.1E-07	7.1E-07	5.9E-07	5.3E-07	5.4E-07	6.3E-07	7.4E-07	6.5E-07	7.2E-07	1.1E-06
Spleen	8.7E-06	5.6E-07	1.4E-05	1.9E-06	1.7E-06	9.4E-07	1.3E-05	1.1E-06	3.2E-06	2.1E-06
Testes	4.4E-08	5.9E-06	6.2E-08	3.8E-07	3.5E-07	2.3E-06	1.2E-07	8.4E-08	1.2E-08	1.6E-06
Thyroid	1.6E-07	3.5E-09	1.2E-07	2.2E-08	2.4E-08	8.4E-09	6.5E-08	2.0E-07	1.1E-06	2.1E-06
Uterus (nongravid)	1.6E-06	2.3E-05	9.2E-07	1.3E-05	6.4E-06	8.9E-06	1.1E-06	4.5E-07	1.0E-07	3.4E-06
Total body	3.4E-06	2.9E-06	3.0E-06	3.7E-06	3.3E-06	3.4E-06	3.4E-06	3.5E-06	3.2E-06	2.9E-06

Target Organs	Source Organs									
			Skeleton							
	Ovaries	Pancreas	Red Marrow	Cortical Bone	Trabecular Bone	Skin	Spleen	Testes	Thyroid	Total Body
Adrenals	4.1E-07	1.2E-05	3.1E-06	1.5E-06	1.5E-06	9.4E-07	8.7E-06	4.4E-08	1.6E-07	3.4E-06
Bladder wall	9.2E-06	1.7E-07	1.1E-06	6.0E-07	6.0E-07	6.6E-07	1.5E-07	6.2E-06	3.6E-09	3.5E-06
Bone (total)	1.9E-06	1.7E-06	7.0E-06	2.0E-05	1.8E-05	1.5E-06	1.5E-06	1.0E-06	1.2E-06	4.0E-06
GI (stomach wall)	9.4E-07	2.8E-05	1.2E-06	6.9E-07	6.9E-07	7.1E-07	1.4E-05	4.8E-08	5.7E-08	3.5E-06
GI (SI)	1.8E-05	2.2E-06	3.3E-06	9.3E-07	9.3E-07	5.7E-07	1.7E-06	4.4E-07	1.3E-08	3.8E-06
GI (ULI wall)	1.8E-05	2.6E-06	2.7E-06	8.7E-07	8.7E-07	5.9E-07	1.7E-06	3.8E-07	1.3E-08	3.7E-06
GI (LLI wall)	2.4E-05	6.6E-07	3.9E-06	1.3E-06	1.3E-06	6.0E-07	7.3E-07	3.4E-06	6.8E-09	3.5E-06
Kidneys	1.1E-06	8.5E-06	2.8E-06	1.1E-06	1.1E-06	8.2E-07	1.3E-05	5.7E-08	4.2E-08	3.3E-06
Liver	6.5E-07	5.7E-06	1.1E-06	8.3E-07	8.3E-07	7.1E-07	1.2E-06	4.1E-08	1.2E-07	3.4E-06
Lungs	7.7E-08	3.3E-06	1.5E-06	1.2E-06	1.2E-06	8.0E-07	3.1E-06	1.0E-08	1.1E-06	3.1E-06
Marrow (red)	7.0E-06	3.3E-06	5.5E-05	7.8E-06	1.5E-05	1.4E-06	2.1E-06	8.1E-07	1.3E-06	4.4E-06
Other tissues (muscles)	2.9E-06	2.6E-06	1.6E-06	1.3E-06	1.3E-06	1.1E-06	2.1E-06	1.6E-06	2.1E-06	2.9E-06
Ovaries	7.2E-03	4.4E-07	3.6E-06	1.0E-06	1.0E-06	5.0E-07	5.7E-07	0.0	7.9E-09	3.6E-06
Pancreas	5.8E-07	1.0E-03	2.0E-06	1.1E-06	1.1E-06	6.0E-07	3.0E-05	6.9E-08	9.5E-08	3.8E-06
Skin	5.1E-07	5.0E-07	8.1E-07	9.0E-07	9.0E-07	2.7E-05	6.3E-07	2.3E-06	1.1E-06	2.0E-06
Spleen	6.0E-07	3.0E-05	1.1E-06	8.0E-07	8.0E-07	7.1E-07	5.9E-04	3.0E-08	1.3E-07	3.5E-06
Testes	0.0	7.1E-08	4.8E-07	7.6E-07	7.6E-07	1.5E-06	6.6E-08	2.5E-03	9.8E-10	2.6E-06
Thyroid	7.9E-09	1.5E-07	8.5E-07	1.0E-06	1.0E-06	1.1E-06	1.1E-07	9.9E-10	4.0E-03	2.6E-06
Uterus (nongravid)	3.0E-05	6.6E-07	2.7E-06	7.2E-07	7.2E-07	5.0E-07	4.7E-07	0.0	7.3E-09	3.9E-06
Total body	3.9E-06	3.9E-06	3.4E-06	3.2E-06	3.2E-06	2.1E-06	3.5E-06	2.9E-06	2.9E-06	3.1E-06

Decay data revised—March, 1972. Reference—MIRD Pamphlet No. 10.

Date of issue, 05-13-75. Reproduced with permission of the Society of Nuclear Medicine (MIRD No. 11).

In the MIRD tables the units of S given for a particular radionuclide of interest must be noted. If S is stated in rads per microcurie-hour, A_0 must be stated in microcuries, and $t_{\frac{1}{2}eff}$ must be stated in hours. If it is necessary to know the absorbed dose in units of grays instead of rads, simply divide the right-hand side of equation 10.19 by 100.

The source organ listed in the MIRD tables for S is the organ in which the radionuclide is distributed. The source organ may be total body. The target organ referred to is the organ for which absorbed dose is to be calculated. The source and target organs may be the same. Table 10.2 gives the MIRD table of S values for ^{99m}Tc, and Table 10.3 gives them for ^{123}I.

Example 10.1

What is the absorbed dose in grays to kidneys for a 4 mCi dose of ^{99m}Tc sulfur colloid? Assume that sulfur colloid has a biologic half-life of 4 hours in the liver and ignore activity in the spleen. From Table 10.2, $t_{\frac{1}{2}p}$ for ^{99m}Tc is approximately 6 hours.

1. $$t_{½eff} = \frac{t_{½p} \cdot t_{½b}}{t_{½p} + t_{½b}}$$

$$= \frac{6 \text{ hrs} \cdot 4 \text{ hrs}}{6 \text{ hrs} + 4 \text{ hrs}} = \frac{24 \text{ (hrs)}^2}{10 \text{ hrs}} = 2.4 \text{ hrs}$$

2. $A_0 = 4 \text{ mCi} = 4 \cdot 10^3\ \mu\text{Ci}$

3. From Table 10.2, S for source organ as the liver (read horizontally to the right; the liver is on the second page of the table, three columns from the right-hand edge) and target organ as the kidneys (read vertically down in the left column of the page), the value 3.9E–06 rads/μCi-hr is obtained. This value means $3.9 \cdot 10^{-6}$; E stands for "exponential," and E-06 is to be interpreted as 10^{-6}.

4. Consequently,

$$D = A_0\ 1.44\ t_{½eff}S$$

$$= 4 \cdot 10^3\ \mu\text{Ci} \cdot 1.44 \cdot 2.4 \text{ hrs} \cdot 3.9$$

$$\cdot\ 10^{-6}\ \frac{\text{rad}}{\mu\text{Ci hr}} \cdot \frac{1\ \text{Gy}}{100\ \text{rad}}$$

$$= 53.9 \cdot 10^{-5}\ \text{Gy} \sim 5.4 \cdot 10^{-4}\ \text{Gy}$$

Example 10.2

What is the absorbed dose in grays to lungs for a 400 μCi dose of ^{123}I sodium iodine? Assume that sodium iodine has a biologic half-life of 17 hours in the thyroid gland. From Table 10.3 the physical half-life of ^{123}I is 13 hours.

$$1.\ t_{\frac{1}{2}eff} = \frac{t_{\frac{1}{2}p} \cdot t_{\frac{1}{2}b}}{t_{\frac{1}{2}p} + t_{\frac{1}{2}b}}$$

$$= \frac{13\ \text{hrs} \cdot 17\ \text{hrs}}{13\ \text{hrs} + 17\ \text{hrs}}$$

$$= \frac{221\ (\text{hrs})^2}{30\ \text{hrs}}$$

$$= 7.37\ \text{hrs} \sim 7.4\ \text{hrs}$$

$$2.\ A_o = 400\ \mu\text{Ci}$$

3. From Table 10.3, S for source organ as thyroid (first page of table, second column from right-hand edge) and lungs as target organ (left-hand column of page), the value of 1.1E–06 rad/μCi-hr is obtained. Hence $S = 1.1 \cdot 10^{-6}$.

4. Consequently,

$$D = A_o\ 1.44\ t_{\frac{1}{2}eff}S$$

$$= 400\ \mu\text{Ci} \cdot 1.44 \cdot 7.4\ \text{hrs} \cdot 1.1 \cdot 10^{-6}\ \frac{\text{rad}}{\mu\text{Ci hr}}\ \frac{1\ \text{Gy}}{100\ \text{rad}}$$

$$= 46.89 \cdot 10^{-6}\text{Gy} \sim 4.7 \cdot 10^{-5}\ \text{Gy}$$

These examples should enable the reader to use the MIRD tables when it is necessary to calculate the internal dose to a particular organ or the total body from a specific radionuclide.*

*It would be impossible to include all the tables that the reader may need. The authors intend only to enable the reader to use the MIRD tables, should the need arise.

BIBLIOGRAPHY

Snyder, W. S., Ford, M. R., and Warner, G. G.: Specific Absorbed Fractions for Radiation Sources Uniformly Distributed in Various Organs of a Heterogeneous Phantom. (To be published as a MIRD pamphlet.)

Snyder, W. S., Ford, M. R., Warner, G. G., and Fisher, H. L., Jr.: Estimates of Absorbed Fractions for Monoenergetic Photon Sources Uniformly Distributed in Various Organs of a Heterogeneous Phantom, MIRD Pamphlet No. 5. J. Nucl. Med. 10 (Suppl. 3):5, 1969.

Snyder, W. S., Ford, M. R., Warner, G. G., and Watson, S. B.: 'S' Absorbed Dose per Unit Cumulated Activity for Selected Radionuclides and Organs, MIRD Pamphlet No. 11. New York, Society of Nuclear Medicine, October, 1975.

Protection from External Radiation

section three

chapter 11

BARRIERS

The establishment of maximum permissible dose limits for radiation workers as well as for the general public allows calculation of shielding requirements for walls, floors, and ceilings of rooms that contain x-ray machines or sealed-source teletherapy machines. Thickness of radionuclide containers can also be determined. Proper shielding design, or barriers, for areas where radiation is present allows use of adjacent areas for other activities. These adjacent areas are designated as either controlled or uncontrolled.

A controlled area is one habitually occupied by persons who are radiation workers and under the jurisdiction of the RPO. An uncontrolled area is one normally occupied by persons who are *not* radiation workers: e.g., the secretary's office and patients' waiting room. However, a radiologist's office and a technician's lounge, provided they are within those areas controlled by the RPO, are considered controlled areas and are also considered occupied by personnel who are allowed the MPD for radiation workers.

The limits for exposure allowed in any area are fixed by the MPD for the type of individual concerned. A radiation worker is allowed an exposure of 50 mSv per year. If this exposure is divided by 50, the approximate number of weeks in a year, the MPD becomes 1.0 mSv per week. Similarly, the MPD for a nonradiation worker (5.0 mSv per year) is found to be 0.1 mSv per week.

In the radiologic and health fields, most of the absorbed dose obtained is due to photon exposure. Since the quality factor for photons is equal to 1.0 and since 1.0 C kg^{-1} (1 exposure unit) is equal to 34 Gy, the MPD may be written in terms of exposure units as 30 μC kg^{-1} per week for controlled areas and 3 μC kg^{-1} per week for uncontrolled areas.

Using the nomogram in Appendix II, the exposure limits are 0.1 R per week for controlled areas and 0.01 R per week for uncontrolled areas.

Protective barriers in the form of added shielding consist of two different types. The thicknesses and composition of walls, floors, and ceilings of rooms designed to protect people in adjacent rooms—including those above and below—from radiation from diagnostic x-ray machines or radiation therapy machines of any type constitute one type of barrier. This first type of protective barrier comes in two varieties depending on whether it is designed to protect against primary beam radiation or secondary radiation. The other type of barrier consists in designing containers to hold radionuclides safely. This latter type of protective barrier is discussed first.

PROTECTION FROM EXTERNAL RADIONUCLIDES

This discussion has been confined to shielding from photons, as a few millimeters of aluminum is usually sufficient to shield from all but the highest-energy beta particles. Remember that, when shielding from beta particles, the shielding material must be carefully chosen so that no photons are produced by bremsstrahlung, as discussed in Chapter 8.

A specific radionuclide may emit more than one energy photon. In addition, each energy photon or photons is emitted at a fixed rate in time. For example, ^{131}I decays via beta decay to one of several excited nuclear states of its offspring, xenon-131 (^{131}Xe). These excited nuclear states lose energy by emitting photons in a variety of ways, which produce photons of many different energies. A photon with an energy of 364 keV is produced 84% of the time. However, with their respective probabilities, all other photons produced must be shielded against as well.

In order to account for all photons emitted by a radionuclide, together with the probability of decay of each photon, a constant known as the specific gamma-ray constant Γ is used. This constant describes exposure rate due to photon emissions of a nuclide at a specific distance from the source; the source is considered to be a point. In the old system of units Γ was stated in Rcm^2mCi^{-1} per hour. In the new system of units Γ is expressed as $\mu Ccm^2kg^{-1}MBq^{-1}$ per hour. Table 11.1 gives values of Γ for some commonly used radionuclides. The point-source assumption is valid provided the source volume is small compared to the distance

Table 11.1

Specific Gamma-Ray Constant Γ for Some Commonly Used Radionuclides

Radionuclide	$\Gamma \cdot 10^{-4}$ $\frac{\mu C\text{-}m^2}{kg\text{-}hr\text{-}MBq}$	Γ $\frac{R\text{-}cm^2}{hr\text{-}mCi}$
^{51}Cr	1.12	0.16†
^{60}Co	92.0	13.2†
^{67}Ga	7.67	1.1†
^{123}I	10.46	1.5*
^{125}I	4.88	0.7†
^{131}I	15.34	2.2*
^{59}Fe	44.63	6.4†
^{75}Se	13.95	2.0†
^{99m}Tc	5.02	0.72*
^{111}In	9.41	1.35*
^{133}Xe	.70	0.1†
^{226}Ra	57.53	8.25†

* Oakridge Dosimetry Laboratory (private communication).

† Jaeger, R.C., et al.: Engineering Compendium on Radiation Shielding, Vol. 1. Berlin, Germany: Springer-Verlag, 1968, pp. 21–30.

Values from Jaeger are reproduced with permission of the U.S. Department of Health, Education and Welfare, Public Health Service, Food and Drug Administration, Bureau of Radiological Health, from the Radiological Health Handbook, rev. ed., January, 1970.

from the source to that point at which exposure rate is being measured.

The exposure rate then for a specified activity of a particular radionuclide at a fixed reference point is given by

$$X_r = \frac{\Gamma A}{d^2} \qquad (11.1)$$

where X_r is the exposure rate, Γ is the specific gamma-ray constant for that particular radionuclide, A is the activity of the radionuclide at the time of measurement, and d is the distance in meters from the source to the position where exposure is being measured.

In Chapter 7 the concept of HVL was thoroughly discussed. This concept is now used to determine exposure rate from a radionuclide. From equation 7.13, replacing number of photons by exposure rate,

$$\frac{X_r}{X_{rb}} = 2^{t/t_{1/2}} = 2^n \qquad (11.2)$$

Here the exposure rate with shielding present is written as X_{rb}. If X_{rb} is then made equal to X_{rp}, the maximum permissible exposure rate for the area under consideration—i.e., controlled or uncontrolled—then the number of HVL's of shielding material necessary can be found by using Table 7.1.

Equation 11.2 can be rewritten as follows, substituting for the value of X_r from equation 11.1,

$$\frac{\Gamma A}{X_{rb} d^2} = 2^n \qquad (11.3)$$

and

$$X_{rb} = \frac{\Gamma A}{d^2} \cdot \frac{1}{2^n} \qquad (11.4)$$

The quantity $1/2^n$ is sometimes known as the attenuation factor, meaning that it represents the fraction of radiation transmitted by a protective barrier between the source and the place where exposure rate is being measured.

The activity of radionuclides decreases with

time, so it is necessary to know the activity at the particular time for which exposure rate is being calculated. If exposure is to be calculated for a given time period, e.g., for a working week of 40 hours, equation 11.4 can be simply multiplied by time only if the physical half-life of the radionuclide is significantly longer than 1 week. If this is not the case, the nuclide must be decayed appropriately for each day or hour, and total exposure obtained as a sum over suitable time periods. Exposure can be written as

$$X_b = \frac{\Gamma At}{d^2} \cdot \frac{1}{2^n} \qquad (11.5)$$

where X_b is the exposure for a time t, which is short compared to the physical half-life $t_{\frac{1}{2}p}$ of the radionuclide. The subscript b is used to designate that a barrier is in place. If no barrier exists, $n = 0$ and $\frac{1}{2^n} = 1.0$. Then $X_b = X$, the exposure when no barrier is in place.

Example 11.1

A radiologist occupies a desk that is 0.5 meter from a 100 MBq source of radium-226 (^{226}Ra), which has a physical half-life of approximately 1600 years. How much shielding must be placed about the source to reduce the radiologist's exposure to the allowable 30 $\mu C\ kg^{-1}$ per week? Γ for ^{226}Ra is 57.5 $\mu C\ cm^2\ kg^{-1} MBq^{-1}$ per hour. Using equation 11.5,

$$X_b = \frac{\Gamma At}{d^2} \cdot \frac{1}{2^n}$$

gives

$$2^n = \frac{\Gamma At}{d^2 X_b}$$

$$= \frac{57.5\ \frac{\mu C \cdot cm^2\ 100\ MBq}{kg \cdot hrs \cdot MBq} \cdot 40\ \frac{hrs}{week}}{0.25 \cdot 10^4\ cm^2 \cdot \frac{30\ \mu C}{kg \cdot week}}$$

$$= \frac{57.5 \cdot 4 \cdot 10^3}{25 \cdot 10^2 \cdot 30}$$

$$= 3.1$$

Therefore, from Table 7.1 a little more than 1.0 HVL of material is required.

PROTECTION FROM PRIMARY X-RAY BEAM SOURCES*

X-ray machines generally are not turned on continuously. Consequently, their output of x-rays is confined to certain definite time periods. Further, the intensity of the x-rays is a function of both tube current in mA and tube voltage in kVp or kVcp (see Glossary). Moreover, x-ray beam direction is an important contributing factor because, as a rule, an x-ray beam travels in one primary direction.

Therefore, in order to describe exposure from an x-ray tube, three standard parameters are used: weekly work load W, use factor U, and occupancy factor T. Weekly work load W for an x-ray generator is the product of average current through the x-ray tube multiplied by maximum expected operating time for the generator in minutes per week. The units for W are, consequently, in mA-minutes per week.

Use and Occupancy

The ICRP has recommended values for U and T as follows: The value $U = 1$ designates full use and is used for the wall, floor, or ceiling routinely exposed to the primary x-ray beam. In most installations the primary x-ray beam points toward the floor; hence the floor of the x-ray room has a use factor of 1.0. The exception is dental installations, where the direction of the primary beam has a use factor of ¼. A value $U = ¼$ designates those walls of the x-ray room not routinely exposed to the primary beam. If the x-ray unit is used routinely in a fixed direction, say, vertically toward the floor, but may be used sometimes in a horizontal fashion (as a fixed or rotating unit), the walls of the room have a use factor of ¼ ($^1/_{16}$ for dental installations). Finally, a use factor of

*Several NCRP reports (listed at the end of this chapter) deal with protection from x-ray and gamma-ray sources as well as with protection in the dental and veterinary medical fields.

$^{1}/_{16}$ indicates occasional use, where rotation of the x-ray machine is possible.

The occupancy factors T are based on type of area for which exposure is being calculated. The ICRP recommends an occupancy factor of 1.0 for any space that is fully occupied. Any type of space where people can congregate—a corridor big enough for a desk, an office, a children's play area—is a candidate for full occupancy. If the area is occupied for less than 40 hours a week, the occupancy factor must be calculated assuming that occupancy of an area for 40 hours a week is equivalent to an occupancy factor of 1.0.

On the other hand, an occupancy factor of ¼ is applied to all areas that are partially occupied. Areas considered partially occupied are corridors within the department, lounge areas, utility rooms, patients' wards and rooms, elevators not routinely used by occupationally exposed personnel, and unattended parking lots. Finally, an occupancy factor of $^{1}/_{16}$ is given to areas that are only used occasionally, for example, closets, stairways, automatic elevators, pavements, streets, and rest rooms not routinely used by occupationally exposed personnel.

Photon Energy

An additional consideration, with respect to reducing exposure from x-ray machines, involves the energy of photons themselves. As the kVp on an x-ray machine is raised, the quality of the x-ray beam changes, that is, the photons have a different energy spectrum. The HVL of the barrier used for shielding depends not only on the material composing the barrier but also on the energy of the photons impinging upon it. In order to account for different energies in the beam, another quantity K is defined. This quantity K gives exposure in units of mC m^2 kg^{-1} mA^{-1} per minute that is expected at a distance of 1.0 meter from the primary beam. K takes into account x-ray tube housing and any other shielding that might be in place surrounding the x-ray tube itself.

Exposure from photons produced by an x-ray machine may then be written as

$$X_b = \frac{WUT}{d^2} K \qquad (11.6)$$

Here the symbol X_b is used to designate a barrier in place. The exposure from x-ray machines must always be reduced to the maximum permissible level in order that areas near the radiation installation be safe for occupancy. Naturally, exposure is always calculated in adjacent areas. Accordingly, X_b is always given the value 30 $\mu C\ kg^{-1}$ or 3.0 $\mu C\ kg^{-1}$, depending upon whether the area in which the exposure is being measured is controlled or uncontrolled. Equation 11.6 is usually written in terms of K as

$$K = \frac{P\ d^2}{WUT} \qquad (11.7)$$

where P has been substituted for X_b and P stands for the maximum permissible exposure per week. The value of K is then found on graphs prepared by the ICRP or the NCRP. Figures 11.1, 11.2, 11.3, and 11.4 are graphs of values of K versus thicknesses of lead (Figures 11.1 through 11.3) or concrete (Figure 11.4), which must then be added to the appropriate wall, floor, or ceiling in order to reduce exposure for a particular kVp value to the allowable limit. These graphs represent empirical data gathered by many different experimenters. The graphs were originally drawn to be used with the old system of units, namely roentgens. Therefore, to use the graphs with the new units, $\mu C\ kg^{-1}$, the value of K obtained must be divided by 258, as noted on Figures 11.1 through 11.4.

Example 11.2

A diagnostic x-ray machine is used at an average of 10 mA for 100 minutes each week at 150 kVp. The x-ray tube is positioned 4 meters from a wall between the radiation room and a radiologist's office. The radiologist sits in his office an average of 20 hours per week. The wall contains 4 centimeters of

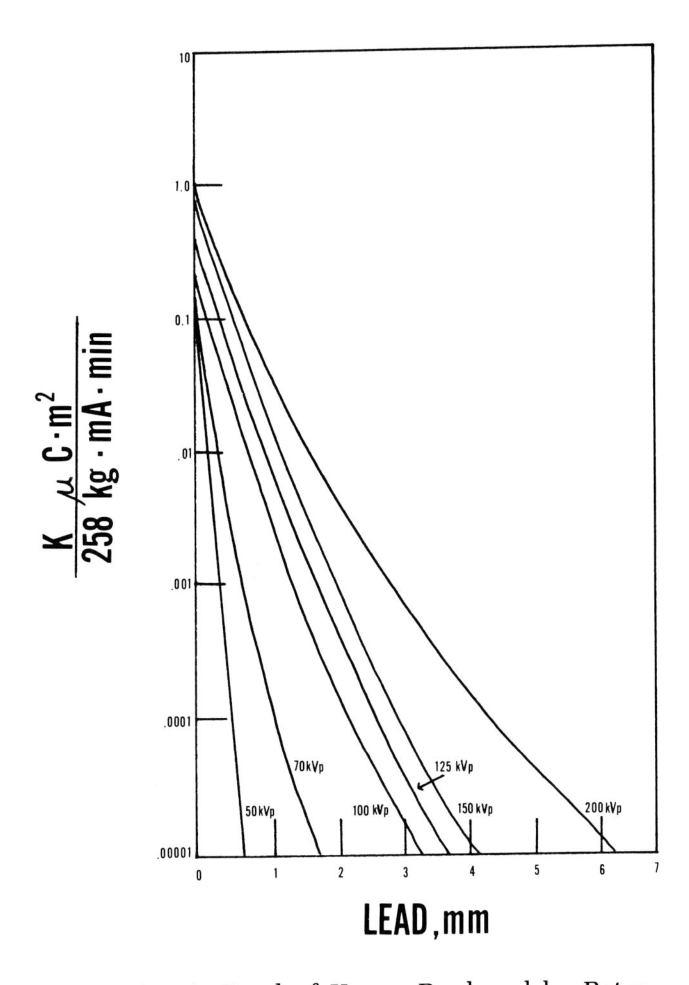

Figure 11.1: Attenuation in Lead of X-rays Produced by Potentials of 50 to 200 kVp. The measurements were made with a 90-degree angle between the electron beam and the axis of the x-ray beam and with a pulsed waveform. The curves at 50 and 70 kVp were obtained by interpolation and extrapolation of available data (data from Braestrup, 1944). The filtrations were 0.5 mm of aluminum for 50, 70, 100, and 125 kVp, and 3 mm of aluminum for 150 and 200 kVp. Direct-current potentials require 10% thicker barriers than those required for the pulsating potentials given above. Note: the y-axis is a log scale. (Reproduced with permission of the U.S. Department of Health, Education and Welfare, Public Health Service, Food and Drug Administration, Bureau of Radiological Health, from the Radiological Health Handbook, rev. ed., January 1970.)

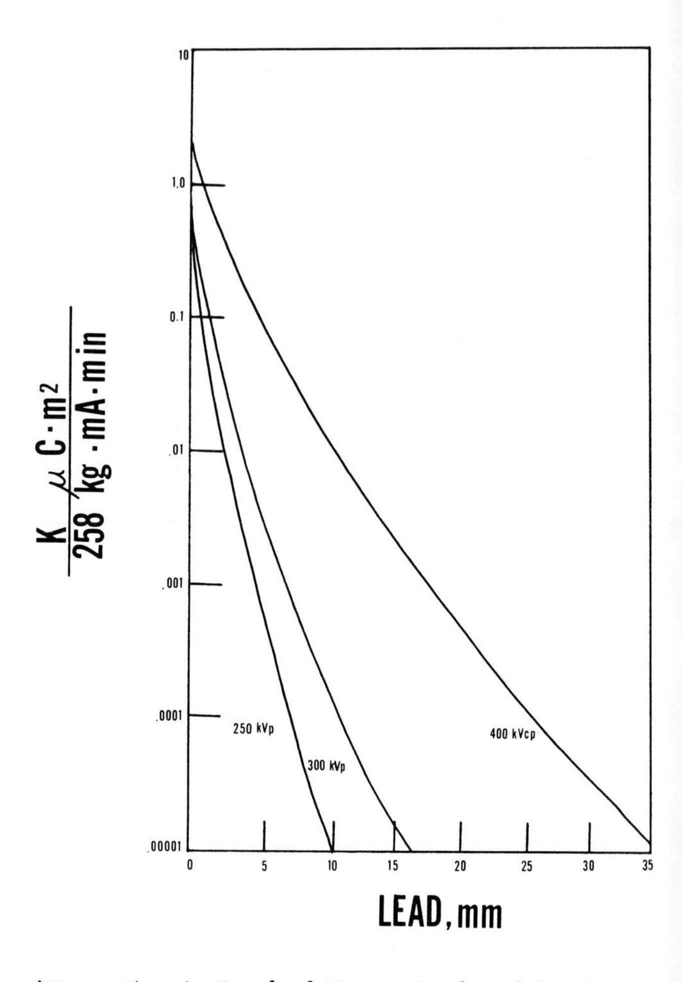

Figure 11.2: Attenuation in Lead of X-rays Produced by Potentials of 250 to 400 kVp. The measurements were made with a 90-degree angle between the electron beam and the axis of the x-ray beam. The 250-kVp curve is for a pulsed waveform and a filtration of 3 mm of aluminum (data from Braestrup, 1944). The 400-kVcp curve was obtained with a constant potential generator and inherent filtration of approximately 3 mm of copper (data from Miller and Kennedy, 1955). The 300-kVp curve is for pulsed waveform and 3 mm of aluminum (data from Trout et al., 1959). Note: the y-axis is a log scale. (Reproduced with permission of the U.S. Department of Health, Education and Welfare, Public Health Service, Food and Drug Administration, Bureau of Radiological Health, from the Radiological Health Handbook, rev. ed., January 1970.)

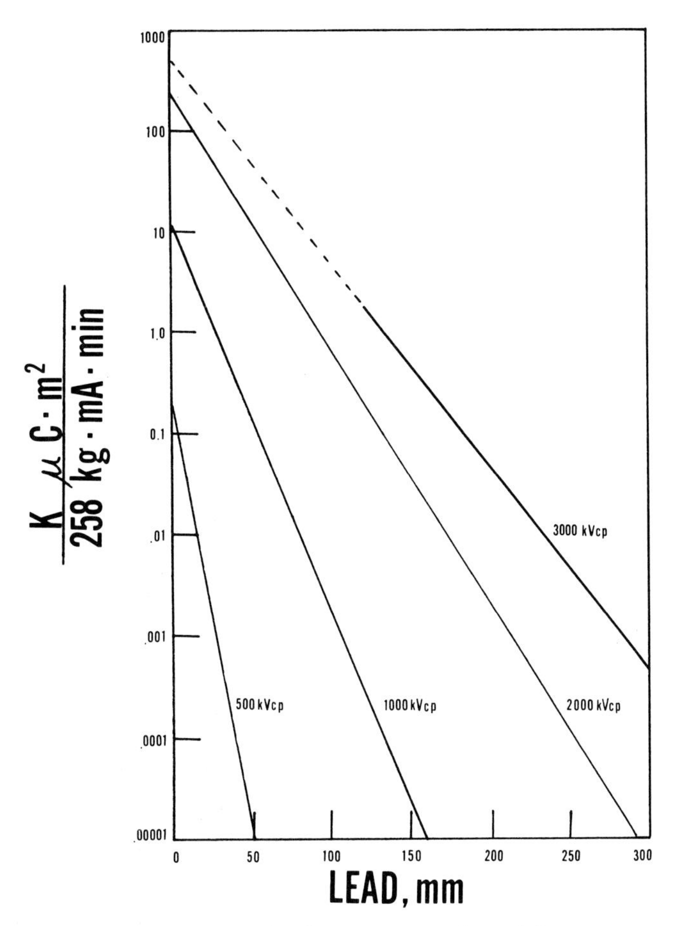

Figure 11.3: Attenuation in Lead of X-rays Produced by Potentials 500- to 3000-kv Constant Potential. The measurements were made with a 0-degree angle between the electron beam and the axis of the x-ray beam with a constant potential generator. The 500- and 1000-kVp curves were obtained with filtration of 2.88 mm of tungsten, 2.8 mm of copper, 2.1 mm of brass, and 18.7 mm of water (data from Wyckoff et al., 1948). The 2000 kVcp curve was obtained by extrapolating to broad-beam conditions (E. E. Smith) the data of Evans et al., 1952. The inherent filtration was equivalent to 6.8 mm of lead. The 3000 kVcp curve has been obtained by interpolation of the 2000-kVcp curve given herein, and the data of Miller and Kennedy, 1955. Note: the y-axis is a log scale. (Reproduced with permission of the U.S. Department of Health, Education and Welfare, Public Health Service, Food and Drug Administration, Bureau of Radiological Health, from the Radiological Health Handbook, rev. ed., January 1970.)

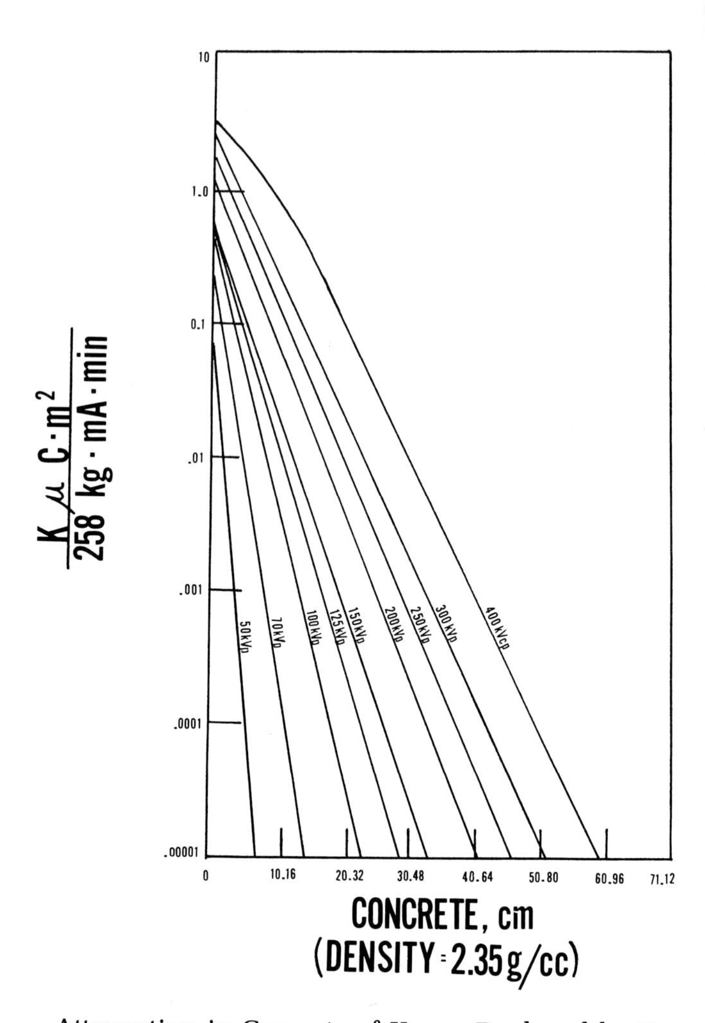

Figure 11.4: Attenuation in Concrete of X-rays Produced by Potentials of 50 to 400 kVp. The measurements were made with a 90-degree angle between the electron beam and the axis of the x-ray beam. The curves for 50 to 300 kVp are for a pulsed waveform. The filtrations were 1 mm of aluminum for 70 kVp, 2 mm of aluminum for 100 kVp, and 3 mm of aluminum for 125 to 300 kVp (data from Trout et al., 1959). The 400-kVcp curve was interpolated from data obtained with a constant potential generator and inherent filtration of approximately 3 mm of copper (data from Miller and Kennedy, 1955). Note: the y-axis is a log scale. (Reproduced with permission of the U.S. Department of Health, Education and Welfare, Public Health Service, Food and Drug Administration, Bureau of Radiological Health, from the Radiological Health Handbook, rev. ed., January 1970.)

ordinary concrete. The primary x-ray beam is directed toward the floor of the radiation room. What thickness of lead must be added to the wall? Using equation 11.7

$$K = \frac{P\,d^2}{WUT}$$

where P equals 30 $\mu C\ kg^{-1}$ since the radiologist's office is a controlled area; d, 4 m; W, 10 mA · 100 minutes per week, which in turn equals 1000 mA-minute per week; U, ¼; and T, 20/40, or ½. Hence

$$K = \frac{30\ \frac{\mu C}{kg\text{-}wk} \cdot 16\ m^2}{\frac{1000\ mA\text{-}min}{week} \cdot \frac{1}{4} \cdot \frac{1}{2}} = 3.84\ \frac{\mu C\text{-}m^2}{kg\text{-}mA\text{-}min}$$

Table 11.2

Equivalents Between Lead and Concrete* at Various X-Ray Tube Potentials

Lead Thickness (mm)	Concrete Equivalents (mm) for the Listed X-ray Tube Potentials			
	150 kVp	*200 kVp*	*300 kVp*	*400 kVp*
1	80	75	56	47
2	150	140	89	70
3	220	200	117	94
4	280	260	140	112
6	—	—	200	140
8	—	—	240	173
10	—	—	280	210
15	—	—	—	280

*Concrete taken as having a density of $2.35 \cdot 10^{-3}\ kgcc^{-1}$.

Reproduced with permission of the U.S. Department of Health, Education and Welfare, Public Health Service, Food and Drug Administration, Bureau of Radiological Health, from the Radiological Health Handbook, rev. ed., January, 1970.

From the 150 kVp curve in Figure 11.1A, 1.2 millimeters of lead are required. The wall already contains 4.0 centimeters of concrete. From Table 11.2 it is found that 1.0 millimeter of lead corresponds to 8.0 centimeters of concrete. Therefore, 0.7 millimeters of lead, or its equivalent in concrete, must be added to the wall.

SECONDARY BARRIERS

It is just as important to shield against scattered and leakage radiation as against primary radiation. Protection from scattered radiation will be discussed first.

Scattered Radiation

It is possible for radiation to be scattered to a location that is not exposed to the primary x-ray beam, always assuming scatter originates at the patient's position. The amount of radiation exposure to a particular location due to scattering depends upon the quality of the x-ray beam (the kVp value), the cross-sectional area of the x-ray beam at the scatterer, and the angle of scattering of the rays. The use factor U is always one for scattered radiation. Provided the location of interest is taken in a direction perpendicular to the primary beam, equation 11.7 is modified in the following ways:*

1. For scattered radiation from useful beams generated at 500 kVp or less,

$$K = \frac{1000 \cdot P \cdot d^2}{WT} \tag{11.8}$$

*The factor 1000 is used in equations 11.8 to 11.11 to account for the reduction in intensity between the scattered radiation and the primary beam. By convention, the ratio of exposure due to primary radiation at the scatterer divided by the exposure due to radiation scattered to a location 1.0 meter from the scatterer is taken to be 1000 provided the location of interest is positioned along a perpendicular to the axis of the primary x-ray beam.

The curves from Figure 11.1 or 11.2 are used for the appropriate kVp of the useful beam. If a 50-cm film-source distance (FSD) scatterer is used, K is divided by 4.

2. For scattered radiation from useful beams generated at 1000 kVp,

$$K = \frac{1000 \cdot P \cdot d^2}{20\ WT} \tag{11.9}$$

3. For scattered radiation from useful beams generated at 2000 kVp

$$K = \frac{1000 \cdot P \cdot d^2}{120\ WT} \tag{11.10}$$

4. For scattered radiation from useful beams generated at 3000 kVp

$$K = \frac{1000 \cdot P \cdot d^2}{300\ WT} \tag{11.11}$$

For K values obtained from equations 11.9, 11.10, or 11.11, the 500 kVp curve from Figure 11.1 or Figure 11.2 is used. Also if the FSD is 70 cm, in each case K is divided by 2.

Leakage Radiation

The ICRP has recommended leakage standards for x-ray tubes as follows: The exposure at 1.0 meter from a diagnostic x-ray tube should be no greater than 30 μC kg^{-1} per hour at a distance of 1.0 meter; and from a therapy x-ray tube, 300 μC kg^{-1} per hour at the same distance. In addition W, the work load per week, is expressed in terms of hours per week the x-ray beam is operating. The use factor U is again set equal to one. In summary then, equation 11.7 is modified to be

$$K = \frac{Pd^2}{30\ (\text{or } 300)\ \frac{\mu C}{kg \cdot hrs} \cdot W \frac{hrs}{week} \cdot T} \cdot \frac{\mu C}{kg \cdot mA \cdot min} \tag{11.12}$$

Here K must be divided by the allowable exposure from the x-ray tube (30 or 300 μC kg^{-1} per hour) and must also be multiplied by the units $\mu C\ kg^{-1}\ mA^{-1}\ min^{-1}$ so that Figures 11.1 through 11.4 may still be used to find the amount of shielding necessary.

A barrier that has been designed to shield against primary radiation is sufficient to shield against scattered and leakage radiation as well. However, if a barrier is designed for scattered and leakage radiation only, barrier thickness is computed separately for each one. If barrier thicknesses computed for each type of radiation differ by more than 3 HVL's, the greater thickness is used for the barrier. If the thicknesses computed for each differ by less than 3 HVL's, the thickness of the barrier is increased by adding 1 HVL to the greater of the two computed thicknesses. Table 11.3 contains HVL thicknesses of lead and concrete for various kVp values.

Example 11.3

A diagnostic x-ray generator is used at an average current of 30 mA for 240 minutes each week at 150 kVp. The x-ray tube is positioned 2.0 meters from a wall between the radiation room and a hematology laboratory (an uncontrolled area). The wall contains 4.0 centimeters of ordinary concrete. For an occupancy factor of 1.0, what thickness of lead should be added to the wall if the primary beam is not directed to the wall? Consider that only scatter and leakage radiation reach the wall.

For the scattered radiation, use equation 11.8,

$$K = \frac{1000 \cdot P \cdot d^2}{WT} \qquad (11.8)$$

P equals 3 $\mu C\ kg^{-1}$ per week because the hematology laboratory is an uncontrolled area. Thus d equals 2.0 meters; W equals 30 mA $\cdot$ 240 minutes per week, which in turn equals 7200 mA minutes per week, and T equals 1.0. Therefore,

$$K = \frac{1000 \cdot \dfrac{3.0\ \mu C}{\text{kg-week}} \cdot 4 m^2}{7200\ \dfrac{\text{mA-min}}{\text{week}} \cdot 1}$$

$$K = 1.67\ \frac{\mu C \cdot m^2}{kg \cdot mA \cdot min}$$

Table 11.3

Half-Value Layers for Lead and Concrete at Various X-Ray Tube Potentials

Attenuating Material	*HVL for Various Tube Potentials (kVp)*									
	50	*70*	*100*	*125*	*150*	*200*	*250*	*300*	*400*	*500*
Lead (mm)	0.05	0.18	0.24	0.27	0.3	0.5	0.8	1.3	2.2	3.6
Concrete (cm)	0.51	1.27	1.8	2.0	2.3	2.5	2.8	3.0	3.3	3.6

Reproduced with permission of the U.S. Department of Health, Education and Welfare, Public Health Service, Food and Drug Administration, Bureau of Radiological Health, from the Radiological Health Handbook, rev. ed., January, 1970.

From the 150 kVp curve in Figure 11.1a, the thickness of lead required is 1.7 millimeters.

For the leakage radiation, using equation 11.12,

$$K = \frac{Pd^2}{30 \frac{\mu C}{kg \cdot hrs} \cdot W \frac{hrs}{week} T} \cdot \frac{\mu C}{kg \cdot mA \cdot min}$$

where P equals 3 $\mu C\ kg^{-1}$ per week, d equals 2.0 meters, W equals 4 hours per week or 240 minutes per week/60 minutes per hour, and T equals 1.0. Therefore,

$$K = \frac{\frac{3.0\ \mu C}{kg\text{-}week} \cdot 4m^2}{30 \frac{\mu C}{kg \cdot hrs} \cdot 4 \frac{hrs}{week} \cdot 1} \frac{\mu C}{kg \cdot mA \cdot min} = 0.1 \frac{\mu C \cdot m^2}{kg \cdot mA \cdot min}$$

From the 150 kVp curve in Figure 11.1a, the thickness of lead required is 2.5 millimeters.

Since the barrier requirements for scatter and for leakage radiation differ (as seen in Table 11.3) by less than 3 HVL's for x-rays generated at 150 kVp, one extra HVL is added to the thickness of lead computed for the leakage radiation. The total amount of lead required is 2.8 millimeters. From Table 11.2, 8.0 centimeters concrete is equal to 1.0 millimeter lead. As a result, 2.3 millimeters lead should be added to the wall.

BARRIERS FOR SEALED-SOURCE TELETHERAPY UNITS

When it is necessary to calculate thickness of barriers for a sealed-source teletherapy unit, equation 11.7 is used once more. In this case, K is replaced by the transmission, or attenuation, factor B. In addition, the work load W is expressed in units of hours per week, and the expression for B is divided by the actual exposure rate X_r in units of $\mu C\ m^2 kg^{-1}$ per hour due to the radioactivity present in the sealed source. Therefore,

$$B = \frac{Pd^2}{X_r WUT} \qquad (11.13)$$

X_r can be evaluated from equation 11.1 as

$$X_r = \frac{\Gamma A}{d^2} \tag{11.1}$$

where Γ is the specific gamma-ray constant for the sealed source. The thickness of the barrier required to provide an attenuation factor B is obtained from graphs prepared from experimental data by the ICRP and the NCRP. Some graphs are shown in Figure 11.5 for those radionuclides most commonly used as sealed sources.*

Example 11.4

What thickness of primary barrier is required for a ^{60}Co teletherapy unit that provides an exposure rate of 13 mC m^2kg^{-1} per hour at a distance of 1.0 meter from the source? Assume that the use and occupancy factors are 1.0 and that the work load is 20 hours per week. The room behind the barrier is 2.0 meters from the source and is a controlled area.

$$B = \frac{Pd^2}{X_r\ WUT}$$

where P equals 30 μC kg^{-1} per week, d equals 2.0 meters, X_r equals 13 mC m^2kg^{-1} per hour or $13 \cdot 10^3$ μC m^2kg^{-1} per hour, W equals 20 hours per week, and U equals T equals 1.

$$B = \frac{\dfrac{30\ \mu C}{kg\text{-}wk} \cdot 4m^2}{13 \cdot 10^3\ \dfrac{\mu C - m^2}{kg\text{-}hr} \cdot \dfrac{20\ hrs}{wk} \cdot 1 \cdot 1}$$

$$= 4.6 \cdot 10^{-4}$$

The thickness of lead required is 14.0 centimeters, as can be seen from Figure 11.5.

*It is impossible to include all the graphs that might be useful. The authors intend only to enable the reader to use these graphs, should the need arise.

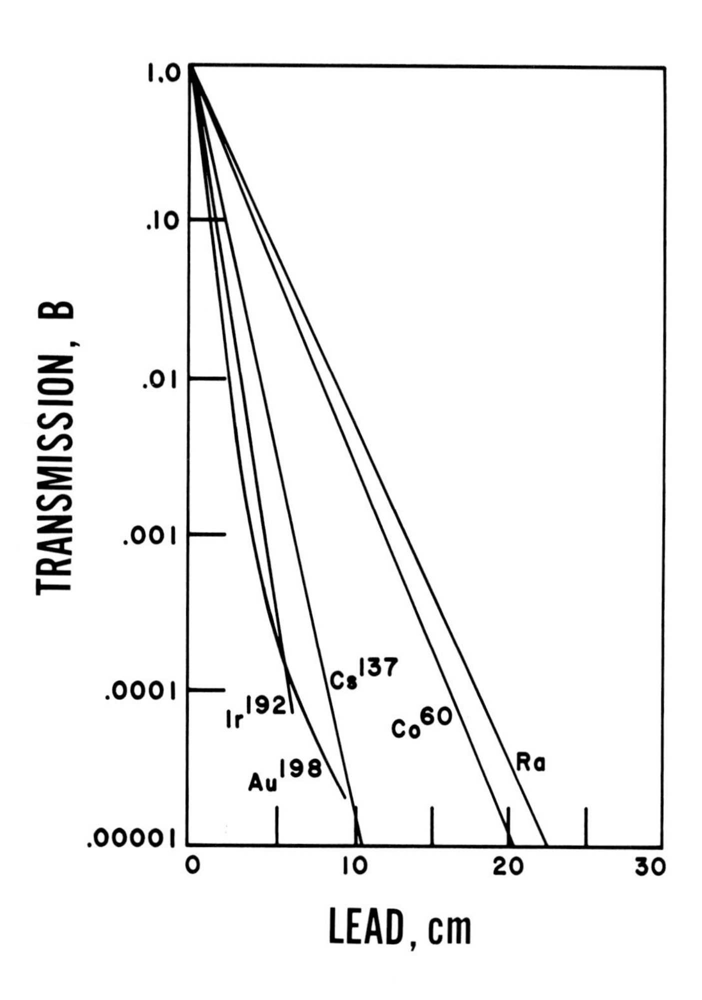

Figure 11.5: Transmission through lead of gamma-rays from radium (data from Wyckoff and Kennedy, 1949); cobalt 60, cesium 137, gold 198 (data from Kirn et al., 1954); and iridium 192 (data from Ritz, 1958). Note: the y-axis is a log scale. (Reproduced with permission of the U.S. Department of Health, Education and Welfare, Public Health Service, Food and Drug Administration, Bureau of Radiological Health, from the Radiological Health Handbook, rev. ed., January 1970.)

COLLIMATION

Beam width, i.e., the cross-sectional beam area, is an important consideration whenever an x-ray or sealed-source gamma-ray machine is used. The width of a photon beam is a function of focal-spot size in the case of an x-ray tube, or of actual size of the sealed source. One method of controlling beam width is by use of collimation.

The finite size of the focal spot or sealed source causes two areas to be of interest: the umbra, or region directly receiving the full strength of primary x- or gamma photons, and the penumbra, which is the region receiving only some photons. A collimator is used to make the umbra a desired size for the purpose of controlling the radiation dose to the patient, particularly to his skin. At the same time, the position of the collimator between the patient and the source is chosen to lessen the penumbra as much as possible.

One limitation exists. Numerous electrons are produced by the interaction of the photons with the collimator. In order to prevent these electrons from reaching the patient, the collimator position should be at least 15 centimeters above the patient's skin. If the photon beam contains a large number of electrons, the energy absorbed by the skin is greatly increased and may result in severe skin reactions.

Sometimes small mirrors are positioned inside the collimator, and these mirrors reflect light from nearby light bulbs. The locations of these mirrors and bulbs are adjusted to provide coincident light and radiation beams emerging from the collimator. This localizer can be used to position patients for diagnostic or therapeutic procedures.

The geometric penumbra, caused by the finite source size (focal spot or sealed source), creates an indistinct border for the radiation field. Figure 11.6 shows the umbra and penumbra on the skin surface and at a depth d within the patient. The width W of the penumbra on the patient's skin is given by

$$W = c\left(\frac{\text{SSD-SCD}}{\text{SCD}}\right) \qquad (11.14)$$

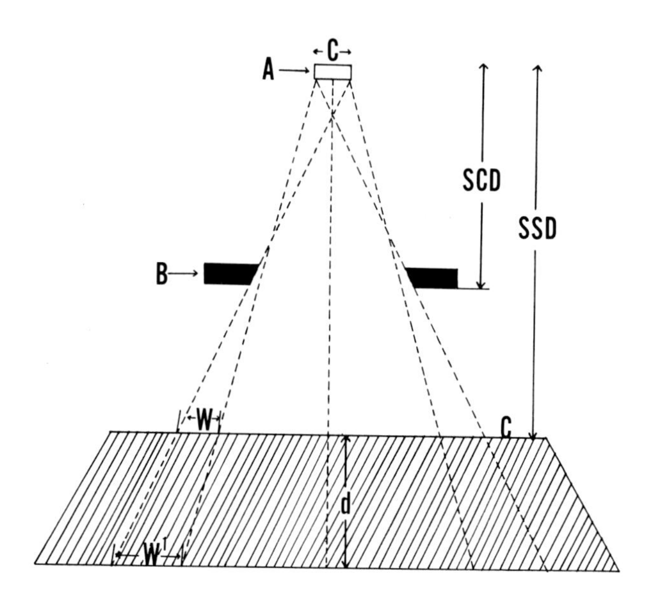

Figure 11.6: Diagram of geometric penumbra caused by finite size (denoted by c) of the photon source (A). The collimator is located at B. The entrance side of the patient's skin is at C. The depth in the patient is denoted by d. The width W of the penumbra at C has widened to W′ at a depth of d. (From Hendee, 1970.)

In this equation, c represents the diameter of the source; SSD is the source-skin distance; and SCD is the source-collimator distance. The width of the penumbra is independent of the radiation field size.

One method of eliminating the penumbra is to place the collimator on the skin. In this case, SSD and SCD become equal, and W is reduced to zero. This practice is undesirable because of the problem with beam electrons, mentioned previously. Sealed sources with high specific activity and small dimensions, such as ^{60}Co, furnish a radiation beam of reasonable intensity and small geometric penumbra.

The width W′ of the penumbra at a depth d within a patient is given by

$$W' = c\left(\frac{SSD + d - SCD}{SCD}\right) \qquad (11.15)$$

The penumbra at any depth within the patient is larger than that on the skin surface.

It is common to define the total penumbra on the surface or at some depth below the surface as the distance between the 10 and 90% decrement lines along the beam edge. These decrement lines are lines through points where the absorbed energy (radiation dose) is a certain percent (e.g., 90, 80, 70) of the energy absorbed at the same depth along the central axis of the radiation beam. The total penumbra on and below the skin should be taken into account when diagnostic or oncologic procedures are being planned.

BIBLIOGRAPHY

Braestrup, C. B.: Industrial radiation hazards. Radiology 43:286, 1944.

Evans, W. W., Granke, R. C., Wright, K. A., and Trump, J. G.: Adsorption of 2 MeV constant potential roentgen rays in concrete. Radiology 58:560, 1952.

Hendee, W. H.: Teletherapy units and high-energy x-ray generators (Chapter 6) and Protection from external sources of radiation (Chapter 25). *In* Medical Radiation Physics. Chicago, Year Book Medical Publishers, 1970.

Johns, H. E., and Cunningham, J. R.: Radiation protection (Chapter XVII). *In* The Physics of Radiology, 3rd ed., Springfield, IL, Charles C Thomas, Publishers, 1974.

Kirn, F. S., Kennedy, R. J., and Wyckoff, H. O.: Attenuation of gamma rays at oblique incidence. Radiology 63:94, 1954.

Miller, W., and Kennedy, R. J.: X-ray attenuation in lead, aluminum and concrete in the range 275–525 kV. Radiology 65:920, 1955.

NCRP Report #33, Medical X-Ray and Gamma-Ray Protection for Energies up to 10 MeV—Equipment Design and Use, 1968.

NCRP Report #35, Dental X-Ray Protection, 1970.

NCRP Report #36, Radiation Protection in Veterinary Medicine, 1970.

NCRP Report #49, Structural Shielding Design and Evaluation for Medical Use of X-Rays and Gamma Rays of Energies up to 10 MeV, 1976.

(Published by NCRP Publications, 790 Woodmont Avenue, P.O. Box 30175, Washington, D.C. 20014.)

Radiological Health Handbook (rev. ed.). Rockville, MD, U.S. Department of Health, Education and Welfare, Public Health Service, Consumer Protection and Environmental Health Service, 1970.

Report of Committee III on Protection Against X-Rays up to Energies of 3 MeV and Beta- and Gamma-Rays from Sealed Sources, International Commission on Radiological Protection. New York, Pergamon Press, 1960.

Ritz, V.H.: Broad and narrow beam attenuation of 192 Ir gamma rays in concrete, steel and lead. Non-Destructive Testing *16*:269, 1958.

Shapiro, J.: Principles of radiation protection (Part II). *In* Radiation Protection. Cambridge, MA, Harvard University Press, 1972.

Trout, E. D., Kelley, J. P., and Lucas, A. C.: Broad beam attenuation in concrete for 50–300 kVp x-rays and in lead for 300 kVp x-rays. Radiology *72*:62, 1959.

Wyckoff, H. O., and Kennedy, R. J.: Concrete as a protective barrier for gamma rays from radium. J. Res., NBS *42*:431, 1949.

Wyckoff, H. O., Kennedy, R. J., and Bradford, J. R.: Broad and narrow beam attenuation of 500 to 1400 kVp x-rays in lead and concrete. Radiology *51*:849, 1948.

chapter 12

External Dose from Photons

The accurate measurement of absorbed dose from an external photon source is fraught with many of the same difficulties encountered before with internal sources (e.g., the specification of organ geometries). Furthermore, as they pass through matter, photons are absorbed or attenuated selectively, depending upon the energy of the photons and upon the density of the material through which they pass. Scattered photons, principally in the form of secondary Compton photons, present a serious complication in the calculation of absorbed dose. In addition, external x-ray sources contain a whole spectrum of different photon energies.

The BEIR report has clearly established that the use of x-rays for medical diagnosis is the largest component of man-made radiation exposure to the general population. As a result, the choice between diagnostic procedures of equal merit is often based on the absorbed radiation dose by the patient. At the same time, oncologic procedures involving photons depend for their effectiveness on delivering a prescribed dose to a specified internal location while at the same time minimizing the radiation dose to surrounding locations.

In this chapter only the basic concepts of external-dose calculations will be elucidated. For a more complete analysis of this problem, the bibliography at the end of the chapter should be consulted.

DOSE IN AIR

In Chapter 5 the exposure from photons is defined in units of C kg^{-1}. The concept of exposure is dependent upon the ionization of air. Since it takes an average energy of 34 eV to liberate one ion pair in air, it is possible to determine the absorbed dose associated with a particular exposure value. Indeed, in Chapter 5 it was found that 1.0 C kg^{-1} exposure was equal to an absorbed dose of 34 Gy in air.

The preceding definitions of exposure and absorbed dose depend upon the ability to construct a standard ionization chamber. This chamber establishes exposure in a cell of free air. Very important to an accurate definition of exposure is the ability to establish electron equilibrium. Recall that in Chapter 5 electron equilibrium is described as the number of electrons entering and leaving the volume in question, being equal for all practical purposes. It is stated there that it can be established only for photon energies below 3 MeV. A calibrated ion chamber, such as a condenser r-meter, can be used to measure exposure at a particular point in space. It is important to remember that a calibrated chamber gives the exposure at its center, which would be recorded if the perturbing influence of the chamber were not present.

DOSE TO A SMALL MASS OF TISSUE EXPOSED IN FREE SPACE

Suppose now that absorbed dose to the center of a small mass of soft tissue Δm situated in free space is to be determined. The mass chosen must be large enough to establish electron equilibrium at its center; hence the mass will have a radius of r_{eq} where eq stands for equilibrium.

As a first attempt to determine energy absorbed by Δm, the mass of soft tissue is replaced by a mass of air, $\Delta m'$, condensed to unit density. The volume occupied by the unit density air is made just large enough to establish electron equilibrium. The masses, Δm and $\Delta m'$, are nearly the same for all tissues of interest in the radiologic and health sciences; thus the equilibrium radii are also the same. In what follows, it has been assumed that $\Delta m = \Delta m'$ and that the electron equilibrium radii are the same.

After exposure to a beam of photons, the dose to $\Delta m'$ and Δm can be determined by placing a calibrated exposure meter at the center of $\Delta m'$. The size of the exposure meter is not important, but the walls of the meter must be thick enough to establish electron equilibrium. The dose to $\Delta m'$ can then be calculated from

$$D_{\Delta m'} = 34 \frac{\text{Gy}}{\text{C kg}^{-1}} \cdot X \text{C kg}^{-1} \cdot A_{eq} \qquad (12.1)$$

A_{eq} is a factor slightly less than 1.0, which gives the fraction of the photon beam transmitted through a thickness r_{eq} of condensed air. If the condensed air mass did not attenuate the photons, the dose to $\Delta m'$ then would be

$$D_{\Delta m'} = 34 \frac{\text{Gy}}{\text{C kg}^{-1}} \cdot X \text{C kg}^{-1} \qquad (12.2)$$

It must be emphasized that equations 12.1 and 12.2 represent different physical situations. Equation 12.2 describes the dose to the air itself, whereas equation 12.1 gives the dose to the center of a small mass $\Delta m'$ of unit density, introduced into air. The introduction of this material gives rise to the factor A_{eq}.

A_{eq} and r_{eq}

This analysis then depends upon determining the value of A_{eq}. In turn, the value of A_{eq} depends upon the thickness r_{eq} of tissue required to establish electron equilibrium. So the main difficulty in obtaining a value for A_{eq} is determining a value for r_{eq}. This latter consideration is made difficult because even a monoenergetic photon beam can set in motion electrons of all energies, from zero to some maximum value. It is standard to choose for r_{eq} the mean range of electrons produced by the photon beam. Consequently, for monoenergetic photons with energies between 200 and 400 keV, A_{eq} has a recommended value of 1.0. For high-energy photons, the value of A_{eq} decreases until it is about 0.90 for photon energies of 25 MeV. The precise value of A_{eq} cannot be determined either experimentally or theoretically. Commonly, a value of 1.00 is used for low photon energies; a value of 0.99, for intermediate energies (^{137}Cs range); and a value of 0.985, for the ^{60}Co−3 MeV Linac range. On the basis of accepted experimental data, workers in this field commonly concur that A_{eq} should be used as just stated and that dosimetry based on these values will not have more than a 0.5% error.

To determine absorbed dose to the tissue Δm exposed in free space, one further step must be taken. For a given photon beam, the energy absorbed is directly proportional to the mass energy transfer coefficient μ_{en} of the stopping material divided by the density ρ of this material. Density is the mass per volume of material. The dose to the medium Δm is given by

$$D_{med} = \left[\frac{34\ (\mu_{en}\rho^{-1})_{med}}{(\mu_{en}\rho^{-1})_{air}}\right] \cdot X \cdot A_{eq} \qquad (12.3)$$

Rigorously, A_{eq} used here should be slightly different from the value used in equation 12.1, which applies to air. It will be assumed, however, that they are the same.

f Factor

The quantity in square brackets in equation 12.3 is very important in dose calculations. It is given the symbol f_{med} and is known as the "f factor":

$$f_{med} = \frac{34\ (\mu_{en}\rho^{-1})_{med}}{(\mu_{en}\rho^{-1})_{air}} \qquad (12.4)$$

Figure 12.1 is a plot of the f factor for monoenergetic photons. As can be seen, for water and muscle, the f factor does not vary much over the entire energy range from 0.01 to 10 MeV. This lack of variance occurs because air, water, and muscle have essen-

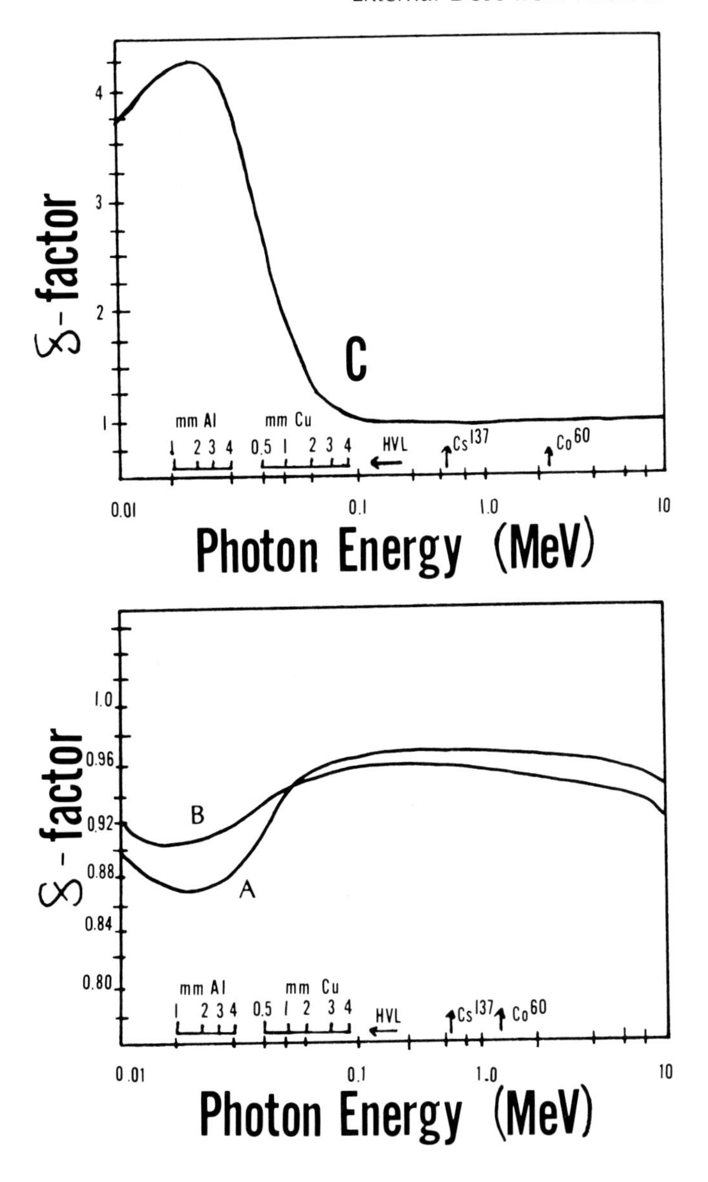

Figure 12.1: (a) The f-factor as a function of photon energy for water, muscle; (b) for bone. The auxiliary scale relates the HVL in aluminum and copper to the energy scale. Curve A represents water; curve B, muscle, and curve C, bone. (From Johns, H. E., and Cunningham, J. R.: The Physics of Radiology, 3rd ed. Springfield, IL, Charles C Thomas, Publisher, 1974.)

tially the same effective atomic number and the same number of electrons per gram; consequently, the quantity $\mu_{en}\rho^{-1}$ is similar for these three materials. Bone, though, has a higher effective atomic number and shows a rapid drop in f for photon energies between 0.04 and 0.1 MeV, where the photoelectric effect ceases to be an important mechanism for stopping photons.

When a material is exposed to a polyenergetic photon beam, such as a diagnostic x-ray beam, it is necessary to weigh the f values obtained from Figure 12.1 by the quantity of photons in the beam having each specific energy. Alternatively, the HVL for the kVp used can be employed to obtain the appropriate f factor. An auxiliary scale for HVL is shown at the bottom of Figure 12.1. Using this scale, an average value f may be obtained directly. The values $\bar{f}$ obtained in this manner are acceptable for absorbed dose calculations.

THE BRAGG-GRAY PRINCIPLE

The determination of dose from a measurement of exposure, as just described, is assuredly the most convenient way of measuring dose; however, this method has two severe limitations:

1. Exposure cannot, strictly speaking, be defined for photon energies above 3 MeV.
2. Exposure methods cannot be used if electron equilibrium cannot be established.

The Bragg-Gray principle, which relates absorbed dose to a measurement of the actual amount of ionization produced in a small, gas-filled cavity in the material, is an attempt to surmount these difficulties.

When a solid material is traversed by a beam of photons, electron tracks are produced, as shown in Figure 12.2. If now a *small*, gas-filled cavity is placed in the material, ionization will be produced in the cavity as well. The Bragg-Gray principle states that, as long as the cavity is so small that it does not alter the number or distribution of electrons that pass through the material, the ionization produced in the

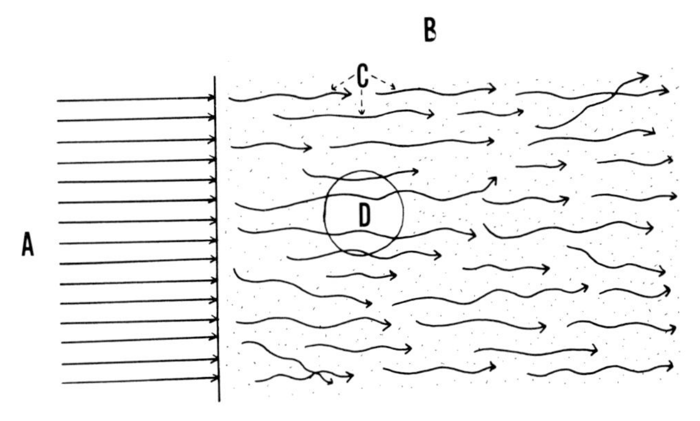

Figure 12.2: Illustration of Bragg-Gray cavity in a medium traversed by electron tracks. The photon beam, A, enters the material, B, and creates electron tracks, C. The small gas-filled cavity, D (size enlarged), does not alter the electron tracks. (Adapted from Johns, H. E., and Cunningham, J. R.: The Physics of Radiology, 3rd ed. Springfield, IL, Charles C Thomas, Publishers, 1974.)

cavity can be related to energy absorbed in the material at position of the cavity. This principle allows determination of absorbed dose at different depths within the material as well as for different densities. It also gives an accurate method of determining experimentally absorbed dose at any particular point in a material such as tissue from any particular x-ray beam.

To find the actual dose to a material, first the energy transferred to the gas in the cavity must be determined. The energy deposited per kilogram of gas in the cavity is given by

$$E_g = J_g \frac{\text{ion pr}}{\text{kg}} \cdot W \frac{\text{J}}{\text{ion pr}} = J_g W \text{ J kg}^{-1} \quad (12.5)$$

$$= J_g W \text{ Gy}$$

The corresponding energy E_m imparted to a unit mass of the material by the same photon beam is given by

$$E_m = S_g^m \cdot E_g \quad (12.6)$$

In equation 12.6 the quantity S_g^m is the mass stopping-power ratio of material to gas. Hence

$$E_m = S_g^m \cdot E_g = S_g^m \cdot J_g \cdot W \qquad (12.7)$$

Each quantity in equation 12.7 must now be examined and its method of determination discussed.

The quantity J_g is determined experimentally. A cavity of known volume filled with a gas of known density and ionization potential is placed within the material. The total quantity of charge produced by the irradiating photons (ion pairs) is measured using a very sensitive charge-measuring device, such as a Keithley electrometer. The volume of a spherical cavity can be determined by measuring its diameter (d) with a measuring device, such as a micrometer, and using the formula $\frac{4}{3}\pi\left(\frac{d}{2}\right)^3$ for the volume of a sphere. Thus

$$J_g = \frac{\text{total charge measured}}{\frac{\text{charge}}{\text{ion pr}}} \cdot \frac{1}{\text{mass}} \qquad (12.8)$$

$$= \frac{\text{total charge measured}}{\frac{\text{charge}}{\text{ion pr}}} \cdot \frac{1}{\text{density} \cdot \text{volume}}$$

Since the charge per ion pair is always equal to $1.6 \cdot 10^{-19}$C

$$J_g = \frac{\text{total charge measured C}}{1.6 \cdot 10^{-19} \frac{\text{C}}{\text{ion pr}} (\rho_g \text{kg cc}^{-1}) (\text{volume cc})} \qquad (12.9)$$

W is the amount of energy in joules needed to liberate one ion pair. Since the ionization potential is usually stated in eV, this quantity must be changed to joules. Consequently,

$$W = \frac{\text{ionization potential (IP)}}{\text{ion pr}}$$

$$= \frac{\text{IP (eV)}}{\text{ion pr}} \cdot 1.6 \cdot 10^{-19} \cdot \frac{\text{J}}{\text{eV}} \qquad (12.10)$$

Table 12.1

Mean Mass Stopping-Power Ratios $\overline{S}^{m}_{air}$

Gamma-Ray Emitter	*Energy of Radiation*	*Polyethylene*	*Water*	*Tissue (Muscle)*	*Polystyrene*	*Lucite*	*Graphite*
^{198}Au	.41 MeV	1.233	1.149	1.149	1.139	1.124	1.013
^{137}Cs	.67 MeV	1.225	1.145	1.145	1.133	1.120	1.010
^{60}Co	1.25 MeV	1.209	1.135	1.133	1.120	1.109	1.002

From National Bureau of Standards Handbook #85.

Consequently,

$$J_g \cdot W = \frac{\text{total charge measured C}}{1.6 \cdot 10^{-19} \dfrac{\text{C}}{\text{ion pr}} (\rho_g \text{kg cc}^{-1}) (\text{volume cc})}$$

$$\cdot \frac{\text{IP (eV)}}{\text{ion pr}} \frac{1.6 \cdot 10^{-19}\text{J}}{\text{eV}}$$

$$= \frac{\text{total charge measured} \cdot \text{IP J}}{\rho_g (\text{volume}) \cdot \text{kg}} \quad (12.10)$$

$$= E_g \text{ Gy.} \quad (12.5)$$

The quantity S_g^m is not so easy to obtain. Many methods for obtaining it have been employed. Table 12.1 gives some mean mass stopping-power ratios ($\bar{S}_g^m$) for the gas air, for several different materials, and for some photon energies. The density of air is approximately $1.3 \cdot 10^{-6}$ kg cc^{-1} at standard temperature and pressure (STP). The absorbed dose to the material is then

$$D_m = E_m = J_g \cdot W \cdot \bar{S}_g^m \quad (12.11)$$

For air as the gas, this equation becomes

$$D_m = E_m = \frac{\text{total charge measured} \cdot 34}{1.3 \cdot 10^{-6} (\text{volume})} \cdot \bar{S}_{air}^m \cdot \text{Gy} \quad (12.12)$$

Example 12.1

A block of lucite is irradiated with photons from a ^{60}Co source. A cavity with a volume of 1.0 cc is placed in the block. Calculate absorbed dose to lucite at the position of the cavity after a charge of 10^{-7}C has been measured by the electrometer. Assume the cavity to be filled with air at STP. $\bar{S}_{air}^{lucite}$ for ^{60}Co is given by Table 12.1 as 1.109. Using equation 12.12,

$$D_{lucite} = \frac{10^{-7} \cdot 34}{1.3 \cdot 10^{-6} \cdot 1.0} \cdot 1.109 \text{ Gy}$$

$$= 29 \cdot 10^{-1} \text{ Gy} = 2.9 \text{ Gy}$$

OTHER DOSE CALCULATION METHODS

Many other methods exist for obtaining absorbed dose from external photon beams beside those described here. One can determine absorbed dose in an extended material by ionization-chamber measurements. It is also possible to measure absorbed dose by calorimetry methods. In addition, various methods of chemical dosimetry have been employed. The use of thermoluminescent devices (TLD's) to measure dose is a more recent development, and film is widely used as well. All of these methods present certain advantages and certain disadvantages; e.g., TLD's can be used conveniently on the surface, but their internal use is limited. That method which is most advantageous for the particular problem at hand should be employed. Depth-dose calculations are of prime importance in the planning of therapy treatments. They are also of importance in choosing diagnostic x-ray procedures.

DOSE IN SELECTED DIAGNOSTIC X-RAY PROCEDURES

The Bureau of Radiological Health has produced both a comprehensive booklet and a small, pocket-sized pamphlet summarizing absorbed dose to selected vital organs and the total body from common diagnostic x-ray procedures. These tables are based on the same model for standard man used in Chapter 10 for internal dosimetry. In fact, the Monte Carlo techniques and geometric considerations developed by the MIRD group have been taken over precisely for these external-dose estimates. The beam quality (kVp technique used) is stated in terms of HVL's of aluminum. The mAs (x-ray tube current, mA, multiplied by the exposure time in seconds, s) is stated in terms of an assumed entrance skin dose of 258 μC kg^{-1} (1000 mR) free-in-air. It is recommended that, at the minimum, anyone engaged in diagnostic radiology obtain the pamphlet and learn how to use it. One table from this pamphlet is reproduced here

Table 12.2

Sample X-ray Doses

Shoulder: Organ dose (Gy) for 258 μC kg^{-1} entrance skin exposure (free-in-air)

Condition: *SID:* 102 cm (40 in.)
(source-to image receptor distance)
Film Size: Full size; see each projection.
Entrance Exposure (free-in-air): 258 μC kg^{-1}

Projection: AP Shoulder (right or left only)
0.254 m · 0.305 m (10 by 12 in.)

Beam Quality	*Dose: 10^{-5} Gy*					
HVL (mm Al)	*1.5*	*2.0*	*2.5*	*3.0*	*3.5*	*4.0*
Testes	*	*	*	*	*	*
Ovaries	**	**	**	**	**	**
Thyroid	11	16	21	26	30	35
Active bone marrow	4.6	6.5	8.5	11	13	16
Embryo (uterus)	***	***	***	***	***	***

Projection: AP Shoulder (both)
0.356 m · 0.432 m (14 by 17 in.)

Beam Quality	*Dose: 10^{-5} Gy*					
HVL (mm Al)	*1.5*	*2.0*	*2.5*	*3.0*	*3.5*	*4.0*
Testes	**	**	**	**	**	**
Ovaries	**	**	**	**	**	**
Thyroid	519	648	748	824	882	927
Active bone marrow	15	21	29	37	47	58
Embryo (uterus)	***	***	***	***	***	***

*No detectable contribution
**$<10^{-7}$ Gy
***$<10^{-8}$ Gy
From Rosenstein, 1976.

as Table 12.2. A sample calculation is done to explicate its use.*

Example 12.2

Use Table 12.2 to calculate absorbed dose to thyroid using two different radiographic procedures.

	CASE A	CASE B
View, projection	AP shoulder; left and right shoulders on separately exposed radiographs	AP shoulder; both shoulders on one radiograph
Field size (at image receptor)	0.254 by 0.305 m (10 by 12 in.) (each radiograph)	0.35 by 0.432 m (14 by 17 in.)
SID	1.016 m (40 in.)	1.016 m (40 in.)
Beam quality (HVL)	2.5 mm Al	2.5 mm Al
Entrance exposure (free-in-air)	65 μC kg^{-1}	65 μC kg^{-1}
Organ of interest	Thyroid	Thyroid
(1) From Table 12.2 the thyroid dose for 258 μC kg^{-1} for HVL = 2.5 mm Al	$21 \cdot 10^{-5}$ Gy (each radiograph) = $42 \cdot 10^{-5}$ Gy (total)	$748 \cdot 10^{-5}$ Gy
(2) The thyroid dose for 65 μC kg^{-1} ($\frac{1}{4} \cdot 258$ μC kg^{-1})	$10.5 \cdot 10^{-5}$ Gy (for standard man where the shoulders are assumed to be 31 cm from the phantom vertex)	$187 \cdot 10^{-5}$ Gy

*When attempting to use the pamphlet, the instructions stated on page 3 should be noted. The beam quality (HVL, mm Al) and entrance exposure free-in-air (μC kg^{-1}) must be determined at the facility. This can be accomplished by direct measurement or by use of one or more of the publications cited at the end of the pamphlet. It is recommended that linear interpolation between listed HVL's be done. When the source-to-image receptor distance (SID) is within 10 inches (25 centimeters) of the listed SID, ignoring this distance difference results in dose variations no larger than 10%. Special precautions are prescribed for calculating absorbed dose to active bone marrow and to testes.

Note the significant reduction (94%) in dose to the thyroid for Case A. Case A can be achieved either by exposing two separate small films or by simply blocking the thyroid area with an appropriate external shield during exposure of the larger film.

CONCLUSIONS

In general, absorbed dose from most radiographic procedures is low. However, the radiation dose from procedures involving fluoroscopy and angiography can be considerably higher. Particular care should be taken when employing these techniques to keep patient dose as low as possible. It is also recommended that radiation worker(s) performing these techniques take as great advantage as possible of the three basic principles of radiation protection: time, distance, and shielding.

Finally, a word should be said about the type of absorbed doses encountered in reconstructed x-ray tomography. The absorbed dose to the patient, generally around 0.02 to 0.05 Gy (2 to 5 rads) uniformly distributed throughout the slice, is high by usual standards employed for diagnostic x-ray procedures. However, in this case as in every case, the medical benefit to the patient must be balanced against expected radiation exposure. As long as this is done, there should be no hesitancy in employing this or any other diagnostic x-ray technique.

The absorbed patient dose from therapeutic x-ray and sealed-source techniques is also high. Procedures, such as rotation techniques, have been developed to minimize absorbed dose to those portions of the patient not undergoing treatment and to maximize absorbed dose to treatment site(s). Treatment planning is, therefore, done on an individual patient basis. As always, the potential benefit to the patient is weighed against possible harmful radiation effects.

BIBLIOGRAPHY

Hendee, W. H.: Measurement of absorbed dose with an ionization chamber (Chapter 10). *In* Medical Radiation Physics. Chicago, Year Book Medical Publishers, 1970.

Johns, H. E., and Cunningham, J. R.: The measurement of absorbed dose (Chapter IX). *In* The Physics of Radiology, 3rd ed. Springfield, IL, Charles C Thomas, Publishers, 1974.

National Academy of Sciences, National Research Council. The Effects on Populations of Exposure to Low Levels of Ionizing Radiations. BEIR Report, 1972 and 1977.

Rosenstein, M. (Ed.): Handbook of Selected Organ Doses for Projections Common in Diagnostic Radiology (Pamphlet). Rockville, MD, U.S. Department of Health, Education and Welfare, Public Health Service, Food and Drug Administration, Bureau of Radiological Health, No. 76–8031, Superintendent of Documents, U.S. Government Printing Office, Washington, D.C., 1976.

Rosenstein, M. (Ed.): Organ Doses in Diagnostic Radiology. Rockville, MD, U.S. Department of Health, Education and Welfare, Public Health Service, Food and Drug Administration, Bureau of Radiological Health, No. 76–8030, Stock No. 017–015–00102–4, Superintendent of Documents, U.S. Government Printing Office, Washington, D.C., 1976.

Appendices

appendix I

The Units of Physics

Physics is an axiomatic system, just like the euclidean geometry taught to all high school students. In geometry, the concepts of point and line are not defined. It is assumed that the student has an intuitive grasp of the meaning of these terms. The concepts of point and line are known as undefined terms.

In physics, the undefined terms are the concepts of mass, length, time, and charge. (Some physicists would not include charge in the undefined terms, but for simplicity, it is included here.) All derived quantities, such as energy, speed, and voltage, are defined in terms of these concepts.

Three systems of units are in general use for describing physical quantities. The English system, because of its limited use, will not be discussed. The other two systems of units are both based on the metric system. The older system is known as the centimeter-gram-sec (cgs) system. The second system is known as the International System (SI) or as the meter-kilogram-sec (mks) system. Each is outlined in Table I.1.

Of the two, the SI is the preferable system, because it is ultimately the simpler. In 1974, SI units were adopted by the International Commission on Radiation Units and Measurements (ICRU), for use in research work and application in radiology. The ICRU has urged that SI units be used completely within as short a period as possible, that period to be extended no longer than 10 years (1984).

Table I.1

Metric Unit Systems

	cgs		*SI (mks)*	
Physical Quantity	*Unit Name*	*Symbol*	*Unit Name*	*Symbol*
Length	centimeter	cm	meter	m
Mass	gram	g	kilogram	kg
Time	sec	s	sec	s
Charge	electrostatic unit	esu	coulomb	C
Energy	erg; electron volt	erg; eV	joule	J
Exposure	roentgen	R	—	Ckg^{-1}
Absorbed dose	rad	rad	gray	Gy
Radioactivity	curie	Ci	becquerel	Bq

appendix II

The Roentgen and the Rad

THE ROENTGEN

Initially, the unit of exposure was defined in terms of the cgs system and was given the name roentgen after W.K. Roentgen (1845–1923), who discovered the phenomenon of x radiation in 1885. In the original definition the roentgen was that exposure of photons which ionized enough air to produce a charge of 1 esu of either sign in a 1 cc volume:

$$1 \text{ R} = 1 \text{ esu cc}^{-1} \text{ (air)} \qquad \text{(II.1)}$$

At STP 1 cc of air weighs 0.001293 g. Hence

$$1 \text{ R} = \frac{1 \text{ esu}}{0.001293 \text{ g}} \text{ (air)} \qquad \text{(II.2)}$$

The equivalence between esu and coulomb is as follows:

$$3 \cdot 10^9 \text{ esu} = 1 \text{ C}, \qquad \text{(II.3)}$$

and

$$1 \text{ g} = 10^{-3} \text{ kg}. \qquad \text{(II.4)}$$

As a result,

$$1 \text{ R} = 2.58 \cdot 10^{-4} \text{ C kg}^{-1} \qquad \text{(II.5)}$$

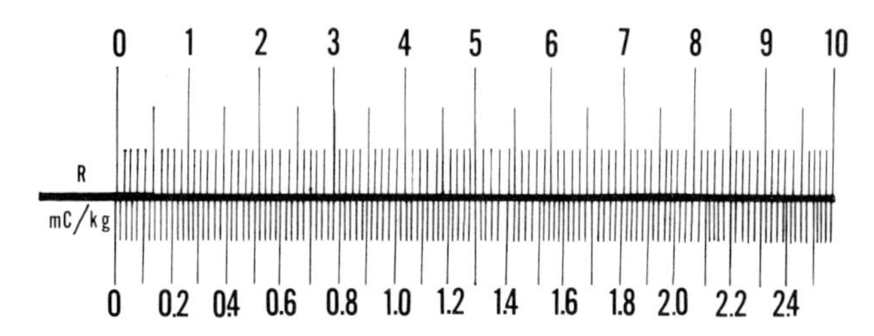

Figure II.1 Nomogram (conversion scale) showing the conversion from roentgens to mC kg^{-1}. (Reprinted with permission from the pamphlet "Units for the Measurement of Radioactivity and Ionizing Radiation" issued by the Metric Conversion Board of Australia, Crows Nest, NSW, 1977.)

This numeric quantity is the one most frequently quoted. Figure II.1 gives a nomogram between R and mC kg^{-1}.

THE RAD

The absorbed dose has been defined in Chapter 5 as the quantity of energy imparted by any ionizing radiation to any material substance per unit mass of that substance. The rad is then defined as 100 ergs of energy deposited per gram of material mass:

$$1 \text{ rad} = 100 \text{ erg g}^{-1} \tag{II.6}$$

The equivalence between ergs and joules is as follows:

$$1 \text{ erg} = 10^{-7} \text{ J} \tag{II.7}$$

Hence

$$1 \text{ rad} = \frac{100 \text{ erg}}{\text{g}} \cdot 10^{-7} \frac{\text{J}}{\text{erg}} \cdot \frac{1 \text{ g}}{10^{-3} \text{ kg}}$$

$$= 10^{-2} \frac{\text{J}}{\text{kg}} = 10^{-2} \text{ Gy}. \tag{II.8}$$

This result is the one obtained earlier:

$$1 \text{ rad} = 10^{-2} \text{ Gy}. \tag{II.9}$$

As a result, if an absorbed dose is quoted in rads, it is only necessary to divide by 100 to express that dose in grays.

THE EQUIVALENCE BETWEEN THE ROENTGEN AND THE RAD

To find the equivalence between the roentgen and the rad, in order to translate exposure measurements into absorbed dose, the procedure is as described in Chapter 5:

$$\begin{aligned} 1 \text{ R} &= 2.58 \cdot 10^{-4} \frac{\text{C}}{\text{kg}} \cdot \frac{10^{-3} \text{ kg}}{\text{g}} \cdot \frac{34 \text{ eV}}{\text{ion pr}} \\ &\cdot 1.6 \cdot 10^{-19} \frac{\text{J}}{\text{ev}} \cdot \frac{1 \text{ ion pr}}{1.6 \cdot 10^{-19}\text{C}} \cdot \frac{1 \text{ erg}}{10^{-7}\text{J}} \\ &= 2.58 \cdot \frac{34 \text{ ergs}}{\text{g}} = 87 \text{ erg g}^{-1} \end{aligned} \tag{II.10}$$

Since

$$1 \text{ rad} = 100 \text{ erg g}^{-1} \tag{II.11}$$

Then

$$1 \text{ R} = 0.87 \text{ rad} \sim 1 \text{ rad}. \tag{II.12}$$

This last equality holds only for photons.

It is common in radiation protection work to use the last equivalence; namely, 1 R is approximately equal to 1 rad. Coupled with the quality factor of 1 for photons, this equation says that an exposure of 1 R to any human person gives him an absorbed dose equivalent of approximately 1 rem when the absorbed dose is measured in units of rads.

As before, it is important to remember that the roentgen is defined only for photons, because it is a unit of exposure. The rad, on the other hand, is defined for all kinds of ionizing radiation.

appendix III

LOGARITHMS

Whenever a number or symbol is raised to a power, such as 2^3, the power is known as the exponent; and the quantity raised is known as the base, or radix. Powers of 10 are quite common in the radiologic and health sciences; 10 constitutes the base.

What are logarithms? The logarithm to the base a of any number b is a number c such that, when a is raised to the power c, it is equal to b.

$$\log_a b = c \qquad \text{(III.1)}$$

which means that

$$a^c = b. \qquad \text{(III.2)}$$

As an example, consider the number 1000, which is equal to 10 multiplied by itself three times, or 10 raised to the power of 3. Then

$$\log_{10} 1000 = 3 \qquad \text{(III.3)}$$

because

$$10^3 = 1000. \qquad \text{(III.4)}$$

When logarithms to the base e (e = 2.7128 . . .) are used, or $\log_e$, it is common to call them natural logarithms and to use the symbol ln. The term "natural logarithms" has come into common usage because many physical laws can be described by equations using base e, and graphs of these quantities are straight lines when the y axis is evaluated in terms of ln.

The rules for using logs are simple and clear. They are the same as the rules for exponents.

1. When two numbers are multiplied together, add the logs:

$$20 \cdot 4 = 80 \tag{III.5}$$

Using ln's:

$$\ln 20 + \ln 4 = \ln 80. \tag{III.6}$$

2. When two numbers are to be divided, subtract the logs:

$$20 \div 4 = 5 \tag{III.7}$$

Using logs:

$$\ln 20 \div \ln 4 = \ln 5. \tag{III.8}$$

3. When a number is to be raised to a power, multiply the log by that power:

$$2^5 = 32 \tag{III.9}$$

Using logs:

$$5 \ln 2 = \ln 32 \tag{III.10}$$

This last equation can also be written as

$$\ln 2^5 = \ln 32; \tag{III.11}$$

hence

$$5 \ln 2 = \ln 2^5. \tag{III.12}$$

4. The log of the base is simply the exponent or power of the base:

$$\ln (e^2) = 2 \tag{III.13}$$

5. When the exponent of the base is a log, then the entire quantity is equal to the value of the log:

$$e^{\ln 2} = 2 \qquad \text{(III.14)}$$

6. Anything that has the exponent 0 is equal to 1, so the log of 1 in any base is equal to 0:

$$\ln 1 = 0 \qquad \text{(III.15)}$$

These simple, yet powerful rules are all that is needed to use logarithms successfully. Table III.1 is a list of natural logarithms.

Table III.1

Natural (Napierian) Logarithms

The natural logarithm of a number is the index of the power to which the base e (2.7182818) must be raised in order to equal the number.

Example: $\log_e 4.12 = \ln 4.12 = 1.4159$.

The table gives the natural logarithms of numbers from 1.00 to 9.99 directly, and permits finding logarithms of numbers outside that range by the addition or subtraction of the natural logarithms of powers of 10.

Example: $\ln 679. = \ln 6.79 + \ln 10^2 = 1.9155 + 4.6052 = 6.5207$
$\ln 0.0679 = \ln 6.79 - \ln 10^2 = 1.9155 - 4.6052 = -2.6897$

Natural Logarithms of 10^k

$\ln 10 = 2.302585$	$\ln 10^4 = 9.210340$	$\ln 10^7 = 16.118096$
$\ln 10^2 = 4.605170$	$\ln 10^5 = 11.512925$	$\ln 10^8 = 18.420681$
$\ln 10^3 = 6.907755$	$\ln 10^6 = 13.815511$	$\ln 10^9 = 20.723266$

To obtain the common logarithm, the natural logarithm is multiplied by $\log_{10} e$, which is 0.434294, or $\log_{10} N = 0.434294 \ln N$.

N	0	1	2	3	4	5	6	7	8	9
1.0	**0.0000**	**0.0100**	**0.0198**	**0.0296**	**0.0392**	**0.0488**	**0.0583**	**0.0677**	**0.0770**	**0.0862**
1.1	0.0953	0.1044	0.1133	0.1222	0.1310	0.1398	0.1484	0.1570	0.1655	0.1740
1.2	0.1823	0.1906	0.1989	0.2070	0.2151	0.2231	0.2311	0.2390	0.2469	0.2546
1.3	0.2624	0.2700	0.2776	0.2852	0.2927	0.3001	0.3075	0.3148	0.3221	0.3293
1.4	0.3365	0.3436	0.3507	0.3577	0.3646	0.3716	0.3784	0.3853	0.3920	0.3988
1.5	0.4055	0.4121	0.4187	0.4253	0.4318	0.4383	0.4447	0.4511	0.4574	0.4637
1.6	0.4700	0.4762	0.4824	0.4886	0.4947	0.5008	0.5068	0.5128	0.5188	0.5247
1.7	0.5306	0.5365	0.5423	0.5481	0.5539	0.5596	0.5653	0.5710	0.5766	0.5822
1.8	0.5878	0.5933	0.5988	0.6043	0.6098	0.6152	0.6206	0.6259	0.6313	0.6366
1.9	0.6419	0.6471	0.6523	0.6575	0.6627	0.6678	0.6729	0.6780	0.6831	0.6881
2.0	**0.6931**	**0.6981**	**0.7031**	**0.7080**	**0.7129**	**0.7178**	**0.7227**	**0.7275**	**0.7324**	**0.7372**
2.1	0.7419	0.7467	0.7514	0.7561	0.7608	0.7655	0.7701	0.7747	0.7793	0.7839
2.2	0.7885	0.7930	0.7975	0.8020	0.8065	0.8109	0.8154	0.8198	0.8242	0.8286
2.3	0.8329	0.8372	0.8416	0.8459	0.8502	0.8544	0.8587	0.8629	0.8671	0.8713
2.4	0.8755	0.8796	0.8838	0.8879	0.8920	0.8961	0.9002	0.9042	0.9083	0.9123
2.5	0.9163	0.9203	0.9243	0.9282	0.9322	0.9361	0.9400	0.9439	0.9478	0.9517
2.6	0.9555	0.9594	0.9632	0.9670	0.9708	0.9746	0.9783	0.9821	0.9858	0.9895
2.7	0.9933	0.9969	1.0006	1.0043	1.0080	1.0116	1.0152	1.0188	1.0225	1.0260
2.8	1.0296	1.0332	1.0367	1.0403	1.0438	1.0473	1.0508	1.0543	1.0578	1.0613
2.9	1.0647	1.0682	1.0716	1.0750	1.0784	1.0818	1.0852	1.0886	1.0919	1.0953
3.0	**1.0986**	**1.1019**	**1.1053**	**1.1086**	**1.1119**	**1.1151**	**1.1184**	**1.1217**	**1.1249**	**1.1282**
3.1	1.1314	1.1346	1.1378	1.1410	1.1442	1.1474	1.1506	1.1537	1.1569	1.1600
3.2	1.1632	1.1663	1.1694	1.1725	1.1756	1.1787	1.1817	1.1848	1.1878	1.1909
3.3	1.1939	1.1969	1.2000	1.2030	1.2060	1.2090	1.2119	1.2149	1.2179	1.2208
3.4	1.2238	1.2267	1.2296	1.2326	1.2355	1.2384	1.2413	1.2442	1.2470	1.2499
3.5	1.2528	1.2556	1.2585	1.2613	1.2641	1.2669	1.2698	1.2726	1.2754	1.2782
3.6	1.2809	1.2837	1.2865	1.2892	1.2920	1.2947	1.2975	1.3002	1.3029	1.3056
3.7	1.3083	1.3110	1.3137	1.3164	1.3191	1.3218	1.3244	1.3271	1.3297	1.3324
3.8	1.3350	1.3376	1.3403	1.3429	1.3455	1.3481	1.3507	1.3533	1.3558	1.3584
3.9	1.3610	1.3635	1.3661	1.3686	1.3712	1.3737	1.3762	1.3788	1.3813	1.3838
4.0	**1.3863**	**1.3888**	**1.3913**	**1.3938**	**1.3962**	**1.3987**	**1.4012**	**1.4036**	**1.4061**	**1.4085**
4.1	1.4110	1.4134	1.4159	1.4183	1.4207	1.4231	1.4255	1.4279	1.4303	1.4327
4.2	1.4351	1.4375	1.4398	1.4422	1.4446	1.4469	1.4493	1.4516	1.4540	1.4563
4.3	1.4586	1.4609	1.4633	1.4656	1.4679	1.4702	1.4725	1.4748	1.4770	1.4793
4.4	1.4816	1.4839	1.4861	1.4884	1.4907	1.4929	1.4951	1.4974	1.4996	1.5019
4.5	1.5041	1.5063	1.5085	1.5107	1.5129	1.5151	1.5173	1.5195	1.5217	1.5239
4.6	1.5261	1.5282	1.5304	1.5326	1.5347	1.5369	1.5390	1.5412	1.5433	1.5454
4.7	1.5476	1.5497	1.5518	1.5539	1.5560	1.5581	1.5602	1.5623	1.5644	1.5665
4.8	1.5686	1.5707	1.5728	1.5748	1.5769	1.5790	1.5810	1.5831	1.5851	1.5872
4.9	1.5892	1.5913	1.5933	1.5953	1.5974	1.5994	1.6014	1.6034	1.6054	1.6074

Table III.1 (Continued)

N	0	1	2	3	4	5	6	7	8	9
5.0	**1.6094**	**1.6114**	**1.6134**	**1.6154**	**1.6174**	**1.6194**	**1.6214**	**1.6233**	**1.6253**	**1.6273**
5.1	1.6292	1.6312	1.6332	1.6351	1.6371	1.6390	1.6409	1.6429	1.6448	1.6467
5.2	1.6487	1.6506	1.6525	1.6544	1.6563	1.6582	1.6601	1.6620	1.6639	1.6658
5.3	1.6677	1.6696	1.6715	1.6734	1.6752	1.6771	1.6790	1.6808	1.6827	1.6845
5.4	1.6864	1.6882	1.6901	1.6919	1.6938	1.6956	1.6974	1.6993	1.7011	1.7029
5.5	1.7047	1.7066	1.7084	1.7102	1.7120	1.7138	1.7156	1.7174	1.7192	1.7210
5.6	1.7228	1.7246	1.7263	1.7281	1.7299	1.7317	1.7334	1.7352	1.7370	1.7387
5.7	1.7405	1.7422	1.7440	1.7457	1.7475	1.7492	1.7509	1.7527	1.7544	1.7561
5.8	1.7579	1.7596	1.7613	1.7630	1.7647	1.7664	1.7681	1.7699	1.7716	1.7733
5.9	1.7750	1.7766	1.7783	1.7800	1.7817	1.7834	1.7851	1.7867	1.7884	1.7901
6.0	**1.7918**	**1.7934**	**1.7951**	**1.7967**	**1.7984**	**1.8001**	**1.8017**	**1.8034**	**1.8050**	**1.8066**
6.1	1.8083	1.8099	1.8116	1.8132	1.8148	1.8165	1.8181	1.8197	1.8213	1.8229
6.2	1.8245	1.8262	1.8278	1.8294	1.8310	1.8326	1.8342	1.8358	1.8374	1.8390
6.3	1.8405	1.8421	1.8437	1.8453	1.8469	1.8485	1.8500	1.8516	1.8532	1.8547
6.4	1.8563	1.8579	1.8594	1.8610	1.8625	1.8641	1.8656	1.8672	1.8687	1.8703
6.5	1.8718	1.8733	1.8749	1.8764	1.8779	1.8795	1.8810	1.8825	1.8840	1.8856
6.6	1.8871	1.8886	1.8901	1.8916	1.8931	1.8946	1.8961	1.8976	1.8991	1.9006
6.7	1.9021	1.9036	1.9051	1.9066	1.9081	1.9095	1.9110	1.9125	1.9140	1.9155
6.8	1.9169	1.9184	1.9199	1.9213	1.9228	1.9242	1.9257	1.9272	1.9286	1.9301
6.9	1.9315	1.9330	1.9344	1.9359	1.9373	1.9387	1.9402	1.9416	1.9430	1.9445
7.0	**1.9459**	**1.9473**	**1.9488**	**1.9502**	**1.9516**	**1.9530**	**1.9544**	**1.9559**	**1.9573**	**1.9587**
7.1	1.9601	1.9615	1.9629	1.9643	1.9657	1.9671	1.9685	1.9699	1.9713	1.9727
7.2	1.9741	1.9755	1.9769	1.9782	1.9796	1.9810	1.9824	1.9838	1.9851	1.9865
7.3	1.9879	1.9892	1.9906	1.9920	1.9933	1.9947	1.9961	1.9974	1.9988	2.0001
7.4	2.0015	2.0028	2.0042	2.0055	2.0069	2.0082	2.0096	2.0109	2.0122	2.0136
7.5	2.0149	2.0162	2.0176	2.0189	2.0202	2.0215	2.0229	2.0242	2.0255	2.0268
7.6	2.0281	2.0295	2.0308	2.0321	2.0334	2.0347	2.0360	2.0373	2.0386	2.0399
7.7	2.0412	2.0425	2.0438	2.0451	2.0464	2.0477	2.0490	2.0503	2.0516	2.0528
7.8	2.0541	2.0554	2.0567	2.0580	2.0592	2.0605	2.0618	2.0631	2.0643	2.0656
7.9	2.0669	2.0681	2.0694	2.0707	2.0719	2.0732	2.0744	2.0757	2.0769	2.0782
8.0	**2.0794**	**2.0807**	**2.0819**	**2.0832**	**2.0844**	**2.0857**	**2.0869**	**2.0882**	**2.0894**	**2.0906**
8.1	2.0919	2.0931	2.0943	2.0956	2.0968	2.0980	2.0992	2.1005	2.1017	2.1029
8.2	2.1041	2.1054	2.1066	2.1078	2.1090	2.1102	2.1114	2.1126	2.1138	2.1150
8.3	2.1163	2.1175	2.1187	2.1199	2.1211	2.1223	2.1235	2.1247	2.1258	2.1270
8.4	2.1282	2.1294	2.1306	2.1318	2.1330	2.1342	2.1353	2.1365	2.1377	2.1389
8.5	2.1401	2.1412	2.1424	2.1436	2.1448	2.1459	2.1471	2.1483	2.1494	2.1506
8.6	2.1518	2.1529	2.1541	2.1552	2.1564	2.1576	2.1587	2.1599	2.1610	2.1622
8.7	2.1633	2.1645	2.1656	2.1668	2.1679	2.1691	2.1702	2.1713	2.1725	2.1736
8.8	2.1748	2.1759	2.1770	2.1782	2.1793	2.1804	2.1815	2.1827	2.1838	2.1849
8.9	2.1861	2.1872	2.1883	2.1894	2.1905	2.1917	2.1928	2.1939	2.1950	2.1961
9.0	**2.1972**	**2.1983**	**2.1994**	**2.2006**	**2.2017**	**2.2028**	**2.2039**	**2.2050**	**2.2061**	**2.2072**
9.1	2.2083	2.2094	2.2105	2.2116	2.2127	2.2138	2.2148	2.2159	2.2170	2.2181
9.2	2.2192	2.2203	2.2214	2.2225	2.2235	2.2246	2.2257	2.2268	2.2279	2.2289
9.3	2.2300	2.2311	2.2322	2.2332	2.2343	2.2354	2.2364	2.2375	2.2386	2.2396
9.4	2.2407	2.2418	2.2428	2.2439	2.2450	2.2460	2.2471	2.2481	2.2492	2.2502
9.5	2.2513	2.2523	2.2534	2.2544	2.2555	2.2565	2.2576	2.2586	2.2597	2.2607
9.6	2.2618	2.2628	2.2638	2.2649	2.2659	2.2670	2.2680	2.2690	2.2701	2.2711
9.7	2.2721	2.2732	2.2742	2.2752	2.2762	2.2773	2.2783	2.2793	2.2803	2.2814
9.8	2.2824	2.2834	2.2844	2.2854	2.2865	2.2875	2.2885	2.2895	2.2905	2.2915
9.9	2.2925	2.2935	2.2946	2.2956	2.2966	2.2976	2.2986	2.2996	2.3006	2.3016

Reproduced with permission of the U.S. Department of Health, Education and Welfare, Public Health Service, Food and Drug Administration, Bureau of Radiological Health, from the Radiological Health Handbook, rev. ed., 1970.

appendix IV

Greek Alphabet

Α	α	alpha
Β	β	beta
Γ	γ	gamma
Δ	δ	delta
Ε	ϵ	epsilon
Ζ	ζ	zeta
Η	η	eta
Θ	θ	theta
Ι	ι	iota
Κ	κ	kappa
Λ	λ	lambda
Μ	μ	mu
Ν	ν	nu
Ξ	ξ	xi
Ο	o	omicron
Π	π	pi
Ρ	ρ	rho
Σ	σ	sigma
Τ	τ	tau
Υ	υ	upsilon
Φ	ϕ	phi
Χ	χ	chi
Ψ	ψ	psi
Ω	ω	omega

Glossary

A

Absorbed Fraction: A term used in internal dosimetry. It is that fraction of the photon energy (emitted within a specified volume of material) which is absorbed by the volume. The absorbed fraction depends on the source distribution, the photon energy, and the size, shape, and composition of the volume.

Absorption: The process by which radiation imparts some or all of its energy to any material through which it passes. (See also Compton Effect, Pair Production and Photoelectric Effect.)

Self-Absorption: Absorption of radiation (emitted by radioactive atoms) by the material in which the atoms are located; in particular, the absorption of radiation within a sample being assayed.

Absorption Coefficient: Fractional decrease in the intensity of a beam of x or gamma radiation per unit thickness (linear absorption coefficient), per unit mass (mass absorption coefficient), or per atom (atomic absorption coefficient) of absorber, due to deposition of energy in the absorber. The total absorption coefficient is the sum of individual energy absorption processes (Compton effect, photoelectric effect, and pair production).

Atomic Absorption Coefficient: The linear absorption coefficient of a nuclide divided by the number of atoms per unit volume of the nuclide. It is equivalent to the nuclide's total cross section for the given radiation.

Compton Absorption Coefficient: That fractional decrease in the energy of a beam of x or gamma radiation due to the deposition of the energy to electrons produced by Compton effect in an absorber. (See also Scattering Coefficient, Compton).

Linear Absorption Coefficient: A factor expressing the fraction of a beam of x or gamma radiation absorbed in unit thickness of material. In the expression $I = I_0e^{-\mu t}$, I_0 is the initial intensity, I the intensity of the beam after passage through a thickness of the material t, and μ is the linear absorption coefficient.

Mass Absorption Coefficient: The linear absorption coefficient per centimeter divided by the density of the absorber in grams per cubic centimeter. It is frequently expressed as

Some of the definitions are reproduced with permission of the U.S. Department of Health, Education and Welfare, Public Health Service, Food and Drug Administration, Bureau of Radiological Health, from the Radiological Health Handbook, rev. ed., 1970.

μ/ρ, where μ is the linear absorption coefficient and ρ the absorber density.

Activity: The number of nuclear transformations occurring in a given quantity of material per unit time.

Adsorption: The adhesion of one substance to the surface of another.

Alpha Particle: A charged particle emitted from the nucleus of an atom having a mass and charge equal in magnitude to those of a helium nucleus, i.e., two protons and two neutrons.

Aluminum Equivalent: The thickness of aluminum affording the same attenuation, under specified conditions, as the material in question.

Anion: Negatively charged ion.

Annihilation (Electron): An interaction between a positive and a negative electron in which they both disappear; their energy, including rest energy, being converted into electromagnetic radiation (called annihilation radiation).

Anode: Positive electrode; electrode to which negative ions are attracted.

Atom: Smallest particle of an element that is capable of entering into a chemical reaction.

Atomic Number: The number of protons in the nucleus of a neutral atom of a nuclide. The "effective atomic number" is calculated from the composition and atomic numbers of a compound or mixture. An element of this atomic number would interact with photons in the same way as the compound or mixture. (Symbol: Z)

Attenuation: The process by which a beam of radiation is reduced in intensity when passing through some material. It is the combination of absorption and scattering processes and leads to a decrease in flux density of the beam when projected through matter.

Attenuation Coefficient: A general term used to describe quantitatively the reduction in intensity of a beam of radiation as it passes through a particular material.

Attenuation Coefficient, Compton: The fractional number of photons removed from a beam of radiation per unit thickness of a material through which it is passing as a result of Compton effect interactions.

Attenuation Coefficient, Linear: The fractional number of photons removed from a beam of radiation per unit thickness of a material through which it is passing due to all absorption and scattering processes.

Attenuation Coefficient, Pair Production: That fractional decrease in the intensity of a beam of ionizing radiation due to pair production in a medium through which it passes.

Attenuation Coefficient, Photoelectric Effect: That fractional decrease in the intensity of a beam of ionizing radiation due to photoelectric effect in a medium through which it is passing.

Attenuation Factor: A measure of the opacity of a layer of material for radiation traversing it; the ratio of the incident intensity to the transmitted intensity. It is equal to I_0/I, where I_0 and I are the intensities of the incident and emergent radiation, respectively. In the usual sense of exponential absorption ($I = I_0e^{-\mu t}$), the attenuation factor is $e^{-\mu t}$, where t is the thickness of the material and μ is the absorption coefficient.

Avalanche: The multiplicative process in which a single charged particle accelerated by a strong electric field produces additional charged particles through collision with neutral gas molecules. This cumulative increase of ions is also known as "Townsend ionization" or "Townsend avalanche."

Average Life (Mean Life): The average of the individual lives of all the atoms of a particular radioactive substance. It is 1.443 times the radioactive half-life.

Avogadro's Number (Avogadro Constant): Number of atoms in a gram atomic weight of any element; also the number of molecules in a gram molecular weight of any substance. It is numerically equal to $6.023 \cdot 10^{23}$ on the unified mass scale. (Symbol: N_A)

B

Barriers, Protective: Barriers of radiation-absorbing material, such as lead, concrete, and plaster, used to reduce radiation exposure.

Barriers, Primary Protective: Barriers sufficient to attenuate the useful beam to the required degree.

Barriers, Secondary Protective: Barriers sufficient to attenuate stray radiation to the required degree.

Beam: A unidirectional or approximately unidirectional flow of electromagnetic radiation or of particles.

Useful Beam (Radiology): Radiation that passes through the aperture, cone, or other collimating device of the source housing; sometimes called "primary beam."

Beam Hardening: The process of eliminating the low energy photons from a beam of x-rays. This process changes the quality of the beam in such a manner that the average energy of the beam increases.

Becquerel: The new special unit of activity. One becquerel equals one nuclear distintegration per second. (Abbreviated Bq)

Beta Particle: Charged particle emitted from the nucleus of an atom, with a mass and charge equal in magnitude to that of the electron.

Biologic Effectiveness of Radiation: (See Relative Biologic Effectiveness.)

Bragg-Gray Principle: The relationship between energy absorbed in a small gas-filled cavity in a medium to energy absorbed (in the medium) from ionizing radiation. The relationship is expressed as $E_m = W \cdot J_g \cdot S_g^m$, where E_m = energy/mass absorbed in the medium, W = average energy needed to produce an ion pair in the gas, J_g = number of ion pairs/mass formed in the gas, and S_g^m = ratio of the stopping power for secondary particles in the medium to that in the gas.

Branching: The occurrence of two or more modes by which a radionuclide can undergo radioactive decay. For example, RaC can undergo α or β^- decay, ^{64}Cu can undergo β^-, β^+, or electron capture decay. An individual atom of a nuclide exhibiting branching disintegrates by one mode only. The fraction disintegrating by a particular mode is the "branching fraction" for that mode. The "branching ratio" is the ratio of two specified branching fractions (also called multiple disintegration).

Bremsstrahlung: Secondary photon radiation produced by deceleration of charged particles passing through matter.

Buildup Factor: The ratio of the intensity of x or gamma radiation (both primary and scattered) at a point in an absorbing medium to the intensity of only the primary radiation. This factor has particular application for "broad beam" attenuation. "Intensity" may refer to energy flux, dose, or energy absorption.

Burial Ground (Graveyard): A place for burying unwanted radioactive objects to prevent escape of their radiations, the earth or water acting as a shield. Such objects must be placed in watertight, noncorrodible containers so the radioactive material cannot leach out and invade underground water supplies.

C

Calibration: Determination of variation from standard, or accuracy, of a measuring instrument to ascertain necessary correction factors.

Capture, Electron: A mode of radioactive decay involving the capture of an orbital electron by its nucleus. Capture from a particular electron shell is designated as K-electron capture, L-electron capture, etc.

Capture, K-Electron: Electron capture from the K shell by the nucleus of the atom. Also loosely used to designate any orbital electron process.

Capture, Radiative: The process by which a nucleus captures an incident particle and loses its excitation energy immediately by the emission of gamma radiation.

Capture, Resonance: An inelastic nuclear collision occurring when the nucleus exhibits a strong tendency to capture incident particles or photons of particular energies.

Cathode: Negative electrode; electrode to which positive ions are attracted.

Cation: Positively charged ion.

Chamber, Ionization: An instrument designed to measure a quantity of ionizing radiation in terms of the charge of electricity associated with ions produced within a defined volume. (See also Condenser r-Meter.)

Air-Wall Ionization Chamber: Ionization chamber in which the materials of the wall and electrodes are so selected as to produce ionization essentially equivalent to that in a free-air ionization chamber. This ionization is possible only over limited ranges of photon energies. Such a chamber is more appropriately termed an air-equivalent ionization chamber.

Extrapolation Ionization Chamber: An ionization chamber with electrodes whose spacing can be adjusted and accurately determined to permit extrapolation of its reading to zero chamber volume.

Free-Air Ionization Chamber: An ionization chamber in which a delimited beam of radiation passes between the electrodes without striking them or other internal parts of the equipment. The electric field is maintained perpendicular to the electrodes in the collecting region. As a result, the ionized volume can be accurately determined from the dimensions of the collecting electrode and the limiting diaphragm. This ionization chamber is the basic standard instrument for x-ray dosimetry within the range of 5 to 1400 kVp.

Standard Ionization Chamber: A specially constructed ionization chamber from which other ionization chambers can be calibrated.

Thimble Ionization Chamber: A small cylindrical or spherical ionization chamber, usually with walls of organic material.

Tissue Equivalent Ionization Chamber: An ionization chamber in which the material of the walls, electrodes, and gas are so selected as to produce ionization essentially equivalent to that characteristic of the tissue under consideration. In some cases it is sufficient to have only tissue equivalent walls, and the gas may be air, provided the air volume is negligible. The essential point in this case is that the contribution to the ionization in the air made by ionizing particles originating in the air is negligible, compared to that produced by ionizing particles characteristic of the wall material.

Chamber, Pocket: A small, pocket-sized ionization chamber used for monitoring radiation exposure of personnel. Before use, it is given a charge, and the amount of discharge is a measure of the radiation exposure.

Charger-Reader: An auxiliary device used for establishing a particular voltage level in an ionization chamber and subsequently for evaluating that voltage level.

Collimator: A device for confining the elements of a beam within an assigned solid angle.

Collision: Encounter between two subatomic particles (including photons) which changes the existing momentum and energy conditions. The products of the collision need not be the same as the initial systems.

Elastic Collision: A collision in which no change occurs either in the internal energy of each participating system or in the sum of their kinetic energies of translation.

Inelastic Collision: A collision in which changes occur both in the internal energy of one or more of the colliding systems and in the sums of the kinetic energies of translation before and after the collision.

Compton Effect: An attenuation process observed for x or gamma radiation in which an incident photon interacts with an orbital electron of an atom to produce a recoil electron and a scattered photon of energy less than the incident photon. (See also Absorption, Pair Production, and Photoelectric Effect.)

Condenser r-Meter: An instrument consisting of an "air-wall" ionization chamber together with auxiliary equipment for charging and measuring its voltage. It is used as an integrating instrument for measuring the exposure of x or gamma radiation in roentgens (R). (See also Chamber, Ionization)

Contamination, Radioactive: Deposition of radioactive material in any place where it is not desired, particularly where its presence may be harmful. The harm may be in vitiating an experiment or a procedure, or in endangering personnel.

Controlled Area: A defined area in which the occupational exposure of personnel (to radiation) is under the supervision of the Radiation Protection Supervisor.

Coulomb: Unit of electric charge in the SI system of units. A quantity of charge equal to 1 ampere second.

Count (Radiation Measurements): The external indication of a device designed to enumerate ionizing events. It may refer to a single detected event or to the total number registered in a given period of time. The term often is erroneously used to designate a disintegration, ionizing event, or voltage pulse.

Spurious Count: In a radiation counting device, a count caused by any agency other than radiation.

Counter, Gas Flow: A device in which an appropriate atmosphere is maintained in the counter tube by allowing a suitable gas to flow slowly through the sensitive volume.

Counter, Geiger-Müller: Highly sensitive, gas-filled radiation-measuring device. It operates at voltages sufficiently high to produce avalanche ionization.

Counter, Proportional: Gas-filled radiation detection device; the pulse produced is proportional to the number of ions formed in the gas by the primary ionizing particle.

Counter, Scintillation: The combination of phosphor, photomultiplier tube, and associated circuits for counting light emissions produced in the phosphors.

Counting, Coincidence: A technique in which particular types of events are distinguished from background events by coincidence circuits, which register coincidences caused by the type of events under consideration.

Counting Ratemeter: An instrument that gives a continuous indication of the average rate of ionizing events.

Cross-Sectional Area (of an x-ray beam): An area in the plane of the beam perpendicular to its direction of travel.

Curie: The old special unit of activity. One curie equals $3.7 \cdot 10^{10}$ nuclear transformations per second. Several fractions of the curie are in common usage. (Abbreviated Ci)

Microcurie: One-millionth of a curie ($3.7 \cdot 10^{4}$ disintegrations per second). Abbreviated μCi.

Millicurie: One-thousandth of a curie ($3.7 \cdot 10^{7}$ disintegrations per second). Abbreviated mCi.

Picocurie: One-millionth of a microcurie ($3.7 \cdot 10^{-2}$ disintegrations per second or 2.22 disintegrations per minute). Abbreviated pCi; replaces the term $\mu\mu$c.

Cutie Pie: An ionization chamber device commonly used for detecting radiation exposure rate.

D

Daughter: Synonym for Offspring. (See Decay Product.)

Decay, Radioactive: Disintegration of the nucleus of an unstable nuclide by spontaneous emission of charged particles and/or photons.

Decay Constant: The fraction of the number of atoms of a radioactive nuclide which decay in unit time. Symbol: λ. (See also Decay Curve and Disintegration Constant.)

Decay Curve: A curve showing the relative amount of radioactive substance remaining after any time interval.

Decay Product: A nuclide resulting from the radioactive disintegration of a radionuclide, formed either directly or as the result of successive transformations in a radioactive series. A decay product may be either radioactive or stable.

Decrement Lines: Imaginary lines drawn through parts where the absorbed energy (radiation dose) is a certain percent of the energy absorbed at the same depth along the central axis of the radiation beam.

Delta Ray: Any secondary ionizing particle ejected by recoil when a primary ionizing particle passes through matter.

Density (Physical): The mass per unit volume of a substance. Usually $kgcc^{-1}$ or gcc^{-1}. (Symbol: ρ)

Detector: An instrument capable of registering the presence of radiation. The two common modes of operation for a detector are:

1. **Mean-level or integrating:** The average effect of the radiation is cumulated over time.
2. **Pulse-type:** Individual radiation interactions are separated or resolved in time.

Directly Ionizing Particles: Charged particles such as alpha or beta particles which cause ionization of an atom without any intermediate interaction taking place.

Disintegration, Nuclear: A spontaneous nuclear transformation (radioactivity) characterized by the emission of energy and/or mass from the nucleus. When numbers of nuclei are involved, the process is characterized by a definite half-life.

Disintegration Constant: The fraction of the number of atoms of a radioactive nuclide which decay in unit time; λ in the equation $N = N_0e^{-\lambda t}$, where N_0 is the initial number of atoms present, and N is the number of atoms present after some time, t. (See also Decay Constant.)

Dose: A general form denoting the quantity of radiation or energy absorbed. For special purposes it must be appropriately qualified. If unqualified, it refers to absorbed dose. (See also Maximum Permissible Dose.)

Absorbed Dose: The energy imparted to matter by ionizing radiation per unit mass of irradiated material at the place of interest. The old unit of absorbed dose is the rad. One rad equals 100 ergs per gram. The new unit of absorbed dose is the gray. One gray equals 1 joule per kilogram. (See also Rad and Tissue Dose.)

Cumulative Dose (Radiation): The total dose resulting from repeated exposures to radiation.

Depth Dose: The radiation dose delivered at a particular depth beneath the surface of the body. It is usually expressed as a percentage of surface dose.

Dose Equivalent (H): A quantity used in radiation protection. It expresses all radiations on a common scale for calculating the effective absorbed dose. It is defined as the product of the absorbed dose and certain modifying factors. (The old unit of dose equivalent is the rem. The new unit of dose equivalent is the sievert (Sv).)

Exit Dose: Dose of radiation at surface of body opposite to that on which the beam is incident.

Integral Dose (Volume Dose): A measure of the total energy absorbed by a patient or object during exposure to radiation.

Maximum Permissible Dose Equivalent (MPD): The greatest dose equivalent that a person or specified part thereof shall be allowed to receive in a given period of time.

Median Lethal Dose (MLD): Dose of radiation that would be required to kill, within a specified period, 50% of the individuals in a large group of animals or organisms; also called LD_{50}.

Percentage Depth Dose: Dose of radiation delivered at a specified depth in tissue, expressed as a percentage of the skin dose.

Permissible Dose: The dose of radiation that an individual may receive within a specified period with expectation of no significantly harmful result.

Skin Dose (Radiology): Absorbed dose at center of irradiation field on skin. It is the sum of the dose in air and scatter from body parts.

Threshold Dose: The minimum absorbed dose that will produce a detectable degree of any given effect.

Tissue Dose: Absorbed dose received by tissue in the region of interest, expressed in rads. (See also Absorbed Dose and Rad.)

Dose Meter, Integrating: Ionization chamber and measuring system designed for determining total radiation administered during an exposure. In medical radiology the chamber is usually designed to be placed on the patient's skin. A device may be included to terminate the exposure when it has reached a desired value.

Dose Rate: Absorbed dose delivered per unit time.

Dose Ratemeter: Any instrument that measures radiation dose rate.

Dosimeter: Instrument to detect and measure accumulated radiation exposure. In common usage, a pencil-size ionization chamber with a self-reading electrometer, used for personnel monitoring.

Dosimetry, Photographic: Determination of cumulative radiation dose with photographic film and density measurement.

E

Efficiency (Counters): A measure of the probability that a count will be recorded when radiation is incident on a detector. Usage varies considerably, so it is well to ascertain which factors (e.g., window transmission, sensitive volume, energy dependence) are included in a given case.

Electrode: A conductor used to establish electric contact with a nonmetallic part of a circuit.

Electrometer: Electrostatic instrument for measuring the difference in potential between two points. Used to measure change in electric potential of charged electrodes resulting from ionization produced by radiation.

Electromotive Force: Potential difference across electrodes tending to produce an electric current.

Electron: A stable elementary particle having an electric charge equal to $\pm 1.60210 \cdot 10^{-19}$ C and a rest mass equal to $9.1091 \cdot 10^{-31}$ kg.

Secondary Electron: An electron ejected from an atom, molecule, or surface as a result of an interaction with a charged particle or photon.

Valence Electron: Electron that is gained, lost, or shared in a chemical reaction.

Electron Affinity: The tendency of a neutral atom to attract a free electron to itself.

Electron Equilibrium: A condition established in a standard ionization chamber whereby the number of electrons entering a specified volume equals the number of electrons leaving that volume.

Electron Volt: A unit of energy equivalent to the energy gained by an electron in passing through a potential difference of 1 volt. Larger multiple units of the electron volt are frequently used: keV for thousand or kilo electron volts; MeV for million or mega electron volts. (Abbreviated: eV, $1 \text{ eV} = 1.6 \cdot 10^{-19}$J.)

Electroscope: Instrument for detecting the presence of electric charges by the deflection of charged bodies. It has two metallic leaves hanging at the end of a very slender vane. When like charges are placed on the leaves, they move apart or repel. As the charge is reduced, the leaves move closer together until they are finally side by side when the charge has been reduced to zero.

Element: A category of atoms all of the same atomic number.

Energy: Capacity for doing work. "Potential energy" is the energy inherent in a mass because of its spatial relation to other masses. "Kinetic energy" is the energy possessed by a mass because of its motion; SI units: $kg \cdot m^2 \cdot sec^{-2}$ or joules.

Binding Energy: The energy represented by the difference in mass between the sum of the component parts and the actual mass of the nucleus.

Excitation Energy: The energy required to change a system from its ground state to an excited state. Each different excited state has a different excitation energy.

Ionizing Energy: The average energy lost by ionizing radiation in producing an ion pair in a gas.

Energy Dependence: The characteristic response of a radiation detector to a given range of radiation energies or wavelengths compared with the response of a standard free-air chamber.

Energy Fluence: The sum of the energies, exclusive of rest energies, of all particles passing through a unit cross-sectional area.

Energy Flux Density (Energy Fluence Rate): The sum of the energies, exclusive of rest energies, of all particles passing through a unit cross-sectional area per unit time (energy fluence per unit of time).

Excitation: The addition of energy to a system, thereby transferring it from its ground state to an excited state. Excitation of a nucleus, an atom, or a molecule can result from absorption of photons or from inelastic collisions with other particles.

Exposure: A measure of the ionization produced in air by x or gamma radiation. It is the sum of the electric charges on all ions of one sign produced in air when all electrons liberated by photons in a volume element of air are completely stopped in air, divided by the mass of the air in the volume element. The old special unit of exposure is the roentgen. The new special unit of exposure is Ckg^{-1}.

Acute Exposure: Radiation exposure of short duration.

Chronic Exposure: Radiation exposure of long duration.

F

Film Badge: A pack of photographic film that measures radiation exposure for personnel monitoring. The badge may contain two or three films of differing sensitivity and filters to shield parts of the film from certain types of radiation.

Film Ring: A film badge in the form of a finger ring.

Filter (Radiology): Primary—A sheet of material, usually metal, placed in a beam of radiation to absorb preferentially the less penetrating components. Secondary—A sheet of material of low atomic number (relative to the primary filter) placed in the filtered beam of radiation produced by the primary filter.

Filtration, Inherent (X-Rays): The filter permanently in the useful beam; it includes the window of the x-ray tube and any permanent tube or source enclosure.

Focal Spot (X-Rays): The part of the target of the x-ray tube struck by the main electron stream.

Frequency: Number of cycles, revolutions, or vibrations completed in a unit of time. (See also Hertz.)

G

Gamma-Ray: Short wavelength electromagnetic radiation of nuclear origin (range of energy from 10 keV to 9 MeV) emitted from the nucleus.

Gas Amplification: As applied to gas ionization radiation detecting instruments, the ratio of the charge collected to the charge produced by the initial ionizing event.

Geiger Region: In an ionization radiation detector, the operating voltage interval in which the charge collected per ionizing event is essentially independent of the number of primary ions produced in the initial ionizing event.

Geiger Threshold: The lowest voltage applied to a counter tube for which the number of pulses produced in the counter tube is essentially the same, regardless of a limited voltage increase.

Geiger Tube: An ionization type radiation detector with a very high sensitivity for photons in the energy range 10 to 1000 keV.

Generator ("Cow"): A device in which a daughter radionuclide is eluted from an ion exchange column containing a parent radionuclide long-lived compared to the daughter.

Genetic Effect of Radiation: Inheritable change, chiefly mutations, produced by the absorption of ionizing radiations. On the basis of present knowledge these effects are purely additive; recovery does not occur.

Glove Box: An enclosure used for working with radionuclides particularly those in the form of powders and volatile liquids.

Gray: The new unit of absorbed dose equal to 1 joule per kilogram in any medium. (See Absorbed Dose.) (Symbol: Gy).

Ground State: The state of a nucleus, atom, or molecule at its lowest energy. All other states are "excited."

H

Half-Life: A general term used to describe the time elapsed until some physical quantity has decreased to half of its original value. Here the concept of half-life will be applied to radionuclides.

Half-Life, Biologic: The time required for the body to eliminate one-half of an administered dosage of any substance by regular processes of elimination. Approximately the same for both stable and radioactive isotopes of a particular element.

Half-Life, Effective: Time required for a radioactive element in an animal body to be diminished 50% as a result of the combined action of radioactive decay and biologic elimination.

$$\text{Effective half-life} = \frac{\text{Biologic half-life} \cdot \text{Radioactive half-life}}{\text{Biologic half-life} + \text{Radioactive half-life}}$$

Half-Life, Radioactive: Time required for a radioactive substance to lose 50% of its activity by decay. Each radionuclide has a unique half-life.

Half-Value Layer (Half Value Thickness) (HVL): The thickness of a specified substance which, when introduced into the path of a given beam of radiation, reduces the exposure rate by one-half.

Hardness (X-Rays): A relative specification of the quality of penetrating power of x-rays. In general, the shorter the wavelength the harder the radiation.

Health, Radiologic: The art and science of protecting human beings from injury by radiation, and promoting better health through beneficial applications of radiation.

Heredity: Transmission of characters and traits from parent to offspring.

Hertz: Unit of frequency equal to 1 cycle per second. (See also Frequency.)

I

Indirectly Ionizing Particles: Particles that cause ionization to occur only after an intermediate interaction producing a charged particle has taken place.

Intensity: Amount of energy per unit time passing through a unit area perpendicular to the line of propagation at the point in question.

Inverse Square Law: A rule relating two physical entities by a particular proportionality constant. This constant is one divided by the square of some other physical quantity, usually the distance between the two physical entities.

Ion: Atomic particle, atom, or chemical radical bearing an electric charge, either negative or positive.

Ion Pair: Two particles of opposite charge, usually referring to the electron and positive atomic or molecular residue resulting after the interaction of ionizing radiation with the orbital electrons of atoms.

Ionization: The process by which a neutral atom or molecule acquires a positive or negative charge.

Primary Ionization: (1) In collision theory: the ionization produced by the primary particles as contrasted to the "total ionization," which includes the "secondary ionization" produced by delta rays. (2) In counter tubes: The total ionization produced by incident radiation without gas amplification.

Secondary Ionization: Ionization produced by delta rays.

Specific Ionization: Number of ion pairs per unit length of path of ionizing radiation in a medium, e.g., per centimeter of air or per micron of tissue.

Total Ionization: The total electric charge of one sign on the ions produced by radiation in the process of losing its kinetic energy. For a given gas, the total ionization is closely proportional to the initial ionization and is nearly independent of the nature of the ionizing radiation. It is frequently used as a measure of radiation energy.

Ionization Density: Number of ion pairs per unit volume.

Ionization Path (Track): The trail of ion pairs produced by an ionizing radiation in its passage through matter.

Ionization Potential: The potential necessary to separate one electron from an atom, resulting in the formation of an ion pair.

Ionizing Event: Any occurrence of a process in which an ion or group of ions is produced.

Irradiation: Exposure to radiation.

Isobars: Nuclides having the same mass number but different atomic numbers.

Isomers: Nuclides having the same number of neutrons and protons but capable of existing, for a measurable time, in different quantum states with different energies and radioactive properties. Commonly, the isomer of higher energy decays to one with lower energy by the process of isometric transition.

Isotones: Nuclides having the same number of neutrons in their nuclei.

Isotopes: Nuclides having the same number of protons in their nuclei, and hence the same atomic number, but differing in the number of neutrons, and therefore in the mass number. Almost identical chemical properties exist between isotopes of a particular element. The term should not be used as a synonym for nuclide.

Stable Isotope: A nonradioactive isotope of an element.

J

Joule: The unit for work and energy, equal to 1 newton expended along a distance of 1 meter (1J = 1N · 1m).

K

Kilo Electron Volt (keV): One thousand electron volts, 10^3 eV.

Kilovolt (kV): A unit of electric potential difference, equal to 1000 volts.

Kilovolt Constant (kVcp): The value in kilovolts of the potential difference of a constant potential generator.

Kilovolt Peak (kVp): The crest value in kilovolts of the potential difference of a pulsating potential generator. When only half the wave is used, the value refers to the useful half of the cycle.

L

Laboratory Monitor: (See Survey Meter.)

Latent Image: The state of developability occurring between the time of exposure of a film to radiation and the processing of that film.

Lead Equivalent: The thickness of lead affording the same attenuation, under specified conditions, as the material in question.

Lesion: A hurt, wound, or local degeneration.

M

Mass: The material equivalent of energy; different from weight in that it neither increases nor decreases with gravitational force.

Mass Numbers: The number of nucleons (protons and neutrons) in the nucleus of an atom. (Symbol: A)

Maximum Permissible Dose (MPD): (See also Dose.)

Mean Free Path: The average distance that particles of a specified type travel before a specified type (or types) of interaction in a given medium. The mean free path may thus be specified for all interactions (i.e., total mean free path) or for particular types of interaction such as scattering, capture, or ionization.

Mean Life: The average lifetime for an atomic or nuclear system in a specified state. For an exponentially decaying system, the average time for the number of atoms or nuclei in a specified state to decrease by a factor of e (2.718).

Mega Electron Volt (MeV): One million electron volts, 10^6 eV.

Milliampere: A unit of current. Generally the current flowing between the filament and anode of an x-ray tube is stated in this unit.

Molybdenum Breakthrough: This term refers to the amount of parent nuclide, molybdenum, contained in an eluted sample of its offspring ^{99m}Tc. 37 kBq (1 μCi) of Mo is allowed per 37 MBq (1 mCi) of ^{99m}Tc eluate. However, no more than 185 kBq (5 μCi) of Mo are allowed per patient dose.

Momentum: The product of the mass of a body and its velocity; SI units, kg · m · sec. $^{-1}$.

Monitoring: Periodic or continuous determination of the amount of ionizing radiation or radioactive contamination present in an occupied region.

Area Monitoring: Routine monitoring of the radiation level or contamination of a particular area, building, room, or equipment. Some laboratories or operations distinguish between routine monitoring and survey activities.

Personnel Monitoring: Monitoring any part of an individual, his breath, or excretions, or any part of his clothing.

Monoenergetic: Having only one energy associated with it.

Monte Carlo Method: A method permitting the solution by means of a computer of problems of physics, such as those of neutron transport, by determining the history of a large number of elementary events by the application of the mathematical theory of random variables.

Mutation: Alteration of the usual hereditary pattern, usually sudden.

N

Natural (Napierian) Logarithms: A system of logarithms using the base e.

Negative Ion: Negative charged ion; commonly termed "anion."

Newton: The unit of force that, when applied to a 1 kilogram mass, will give it an acceleration of 1 meter per second per second. (1N = 1 kg · 1m ·1s^{-2}).

Nomogram: Conversion scale between two sets of units.

Nonionizing Radiation: Radiation that does not cause ionization when it interacts with matter.

Nucleon: Common name for a constituent particle of the nucleus. Commonly applied to a proton or neutron.

Nucleus (Nuclear): That part of an atom in which the total positive electric charge and most of the mass is concentrated.

Nuclide: A species of atom characterized by the constitution of its nucleus. The nuclear constitution is specified by the number of protons (Z), number of neutrons (N), and energy content; or, alternatively, by the atomic number (Z), mass number A = (N + Z), and atomic mass. To be regarded as a distinct nuclide, the atom must be capable of existing for a measurable time. Thus nuclear isomers are separate nuclides, whereas promptly decaying excited nuclear states and unstable intermediates in nuclear reactions are not so considered.

O

Oncology: Preferred name for radiation therapy. (See Therapy, Radiation Therapy.)

Offspring: (See Decay Product.) Synonym for Daughter.

P

Pair Production: An absorption process for x and gamma radiation in which the incident photon is annihilated in the vicinity of the nucleus of the absorbing atom, with subsequent production of an electron and positron pair. This reaction only occurs for incident photon energies exceeding 1.02 MeV. (See also Absorption, Compton Effect, and Photoelectric Effect.)

Parent: A radionuclide that, upon disintegration, yields a specific nuclide—either directly or as a later member of a radioactive series.

Path, Mean Free: Average distance a particle travels between collisions.

Penumbra: The region within the beam receiving only some of the primary x- or gamma-ray photons.

Periodic Table: An arrangement of chemical elements in order of increasing atomic number. Elements of similar properties are placed one under the other, yielding groups and families of elements. Within each group, a gradation of chemical and physical properties exists but, in general, chemical behavior is similar. From group to group, however, a progressive shift of chemical behavior occurs from one end of the table to the other.

Personnel Monitor: A dosimeter (usually a film badge, thermoluminescent device, or ionization chamber) used for determining the exposure to an individual. Such monitoring is required for all persons who are radiation workers.

Phantom: A volume of material approximating as closely as possible the density and effective atomic number of tissue. Ideally a phantom should behave in respect to absorption of radiation in the same manner as tissue. Radiation dose measurements made within or on a phantom provide a means of determining the radiation dose within or on a body under similar exposure conditions. Some materials commonly used in phantoms are water, Masonite, pressed wood, and beeswax.

Photoelectric Effect: Process by which a photon ejects an electron from an atom. All energy of the photon is absorbed in ejecting the electron and in imparting kinetic energy to it. (See also Absorption, Compton Effect, and Pair Production.)

Photon: A quantity of electromagnetic energy (E) whose value in joules is the product of its frequency (ν) in hertz and Planck constant (h). The equation is: $E = h\nu$. (See also Radiation.)

Pig: A lead-lined container used for storing radionuclides.

Planck Constant: A natural constant of proportionality (h) relating the frequency of a quantum of energy to the total energy of the quantum.

$$h = \frac{E}{\nu} = 6.6256 \times 10^{-34} \text{ J s.}$$

Plateau: As applied to radiation detector chambers, the level portion of the counting rate-voltage curve where changes in operating voltage introduce minimum changes in the counting rate.

Positive Ion: Positively charged ion; commonly called cation.

Positron: Particle equal in mass to the electron and having an equal but positive charge.

Potential Difference: Work required to carry a unit positive charge from one point to another.

Power, Stopping: A measure of the effect of a substance upon the kinetic energy of a charged particle passing through it.

Proportional Region: Voltage range in which the gas amplification is greater than one, and in which the charge collected is proportional to the charge produced by the initial ionizing event.

Proton: Elementary nuclear particle with a positive electric charge equal numerically to the charge of the electron and a mass of 1.007277 mass units.

Q

Quality (Radiology): The characteristic spectral-energy distribution of x radiation. It is usually expressed in terms of effective wavelengths of half-value layers of a suitable material; e.g., up to 20 kV, cellophane; 20 to 120 kVp, aluminum; 120 to 400 kVp, copper; over 400 kVp, tin.

Quality Factor (Q): The linear-energy-transfer-dependent factor by which absorbed doses are multiplied to obtain (for radiation protection purposes) a quantity that expresses—on a common scale for all ionizing radiations—the effectiveness of the absorbed dose.

Quantum: An observable quantity is said to be "quantized" when its magnitude is, in some or all of its range, restricted to a discrete set of values. If the magnitude of the quantity is always a multiple of a definite unit, that unit is called the quantum (of the quantity). For example, the quantum or unit of orbital angular momentum is h, and the quantum of energy of electromagnetic radiation of frequency ν is $h\nu$. In field theories, a field (or the field equations) is quantized by application of a proper quantum mechanical procedure. This quantization results in the existence of a fundamental field particle, which may be called the field quantum. Thus, the photon is a quantum of the electromagnetic field, and in nuclear field theories the meson is considered the quantum of the nuclear field.

Quantum Theory: The concept that energy is radiated intermittently in units of definite magnitude called quanta, and absorbed in a like manner.

Quenching: The process of inhibiting continuous or multiple discharge in a counter tube which uses gas amplification.

Quenching Vapor: Polyatomic gas used in Geiger-Müller counters to quench or extinguish avalanche ionization.

R

Rad: The old unit of absorbed dose equal to 0.01 joule per kilogram in any medium. (See also Absorbed Dose and Tissue Dose)

Radiation: (1) The emission and propagation of energy through space or through a material medium in the form of waves; for instance, the emission and propagation of electromagnetic waves, or of sound and elastic waves. (2) The energy propagated through space or through a material medium as waves; for example, energy in the form of electromagnetic waves or elastic waves. The term radiation or radiant energy, when unqualified, usually refers to electromagnetic radiation. Such radiation commonly is classified, according to frequency, as hertzian, infrared, visible (light), ultraviolet, x-ray, and gamma-ray. (See also Photon.) (3) By extension, corpuscular emissions, such as alpha and beta radiation, or rays of mixed or unknown type, as cosmic radiation.

Annihilation Radiation: Photons produced when an electron and a positron unite and cease to exist. The annihilation of a positron-electron pair results in the production of two photons, each of 0.51 MeV energy.

Background Radiation: Radiation arising from radioactive material other than the one directly under consideration. Background radiation due to cosmic rays and natural radioactivity is always present. Background radiation may also be due to the presence of radioactive substances in other parts of the building or in the building material itself.

Characteristic (Discrete) Radiation: Radiation originating from an atom after removal of an electron or excitation of the nucleus. The wavelength of the emitted radiation is specific, depending only on the nuclide and particular energy levels involved.

External Radiation: Radiation from a source outside the body—the radiation must penetrate the skin.

Internal Radiation: Radiation from a source within the body (as a result of deposition of radionuclides in body tissues.)

Ionizing Radiation: Any electromagnetic or particulate radiation capable of producing ions, directly or indirectly, in its passage through matter.

Leakage (Direct) Radiation: All radiation coming from the source housing except the useful beam.

Monochromatic Radiation: Electromagnetic radiation of a single wavelength, or radiation in which all the photons have the same energy.

Monoenergetic Radiation: Radiation of a given type (e.g., alpha, beta, neutron, gamma) in which all particles or photons originate with and have the same energy.

Primary Radiation: The useful beam of an x-ray tube.

Scattered Radiation: Radiation that, during its passage through a substance, has been deviated in direction. It may also have been modified by a decrease in energy.

Secondary Radiation: Radiation resulting from absorption of other radiation in matter. It may be either electromagnetic or particulate.

Radioactivity: The property of certain nuclides of (1) spontaneously emitting particles or gamma radiation or (2) emitting x radiation following orbital electron capture or (3) undergoing spontaneous fission.

Artificial Radioactivity: Man-made radioactivity produced by particle bombardment or electromagnetic irradiation, as opposed to natural radioactivity.

Induced Radioactivity: Radioactivity produced in a substance after bombardment with neutrons or other particles. The resulting activity is "natural radioactivity" if formed by nuclear reactions occurring in nature, and "artificial radioactivity" if the reactions are caused by man.

Natural Radioactivity: The property of radioactivity exhibited by more than 50 naturally occurring radionuclides.

Radiography: The making of shadow images on photographic emulsion by the action of ionizing radiation. The image is the result of the differential attenuation of the radiation in its passage through the object being radiographed.

Radiology: That branch of medicine which deals with the diagnostic and therapeutic applications of radiant energy, including x-rays and radionuclides.

Radionuclide: A nuclide that displays the property of radioactivity.

Radiopharmaceutical: A pharmaceutical compound that has been tagged with a radionuclide.

Range: The depth in any material measured from the entrance of an ionizing particle to the stopping position of that particle after it has lost all of its energy.

Reaction (Nuclear): An induced nuclear disintegration, i.e., a process occurring when a nucleus comes in contact with a photon, an elementary particle, or another nucleus. In many cases the reaction can be represented by the symbolic equation: $X + a \rightarrow Y + b$ or, in abbreviated form, X(a,b) Y. X is the target nucleus, a is the incident particle or photon, b is an emitted particle or photon, and Y is the product nucleus.

Recombination: The return of an

ionized atom or molecule to the neutral state.

Relative Biologic Effectiveness (RBE): The RBE is a factor used to compare the biologic effectiveness of absorbed radiation doses (i.e., rads) due to different types of ionizing radiation; more specifically, it is the experimentally determined ratio of an absorbed dose of radiation in question to the absorbed dose of a reference radiation required to produce an identical biologic effect in a particular experimental organism or tissue. NOTE: This term should not be used in radiation protection. (See also Quality Factor.)

Rem: A special unit of dose equivalent. The dose equivalent in rems is numerically equal to the absorbed dose in rads multiplied by the quality factor, the distribution factor, and any other necessary modifying factors.

Resolving Time, Counter: The minimum time interval between two distinct events which will permit both to be counted. It may refer to an electronic circuit, a mechanical indicating device, or a counter tube.

Rest Mass: The intrinsic mass of any physical entity; the mass possessed by that entity apart from any motion it may have.

Roentgen (R): The special unit of exposure. One roentgen equals $2.58 \cdot 10^{-4}$ coulomb per kilogram of air. (See also Exposure.)

Roentgenography: Radiography by means of x-rays.

Roentgenology: That part of radiology which pertains to x-rays.

Roentgen Rays: x-rays.

S

Scattering: Change of direction of subatomic particles or photons as a result of a collision or interaction.

Coherent Scattering: Scattering of photons or particles in which definite phase relationships exist between the incoming and the scattered waves. Coherence manifests itself in the interference between the waves scattered by two or more scattering centers. An example is the Bragg scattering of x-rays and neutrons by the regularly spaced atoms in a crystal, for which constructive interference occurs only at definite angles, called "Bragg angles."

Compton Scattering: The scattering of a photon by an electron. Part of the energy and momentum of the incident photon is transferred to the electron, and the remaining part is carried away by the scattered photon.

Elastic Scattering: Scattering caused by elastic collisions, and therefore conserving kinetic energy of the system. Rayleigh scattering is a form of elastic scattering.

Incoherent Scattering: Scattering of photons or particles in which the scattering elements act independently of one another; no definite phase relationships exist among the different parts of the scattered beam. The intensity of the scattered radiation at any point is obtained by adding the intensities of the scattered radiation reaching this point from the independent scattering elements.

Inelastic Scattering: The type of scattering that results in the nucleus being left in an excited state and the total kinetic energy being decreased.

Scattering Coefficient, Compton: That fractional decrease in the energy of a beam of x or gamma radiation in an absorber due to the energy carried off by scattered photons in the Compton effect. (See also Compton Absorption Coefficient.)

Sealed Source: A radioactive source sealed in an impervious container which has sufficient mechanical strength to prevent contact with and dispersion of the radioactive material under the conditions of use and wear for which it was designed.

Series, Radioactive: A succession of nuclides, each of which transforms by radioactive disintegration into the next until a stable nuclide results. The first member is called the "parent," the intermediate members are called "daughters," and the final stable member is called the "end product."

Shield: A body of material used to prevent or reduce the passage of particles or radiation. A shield may be designated according to what it is intended to absorb (as a gamma-ray shield or neutron shield), or according to the kind of protection it is intended to give (as a background, biologic, or thermal shield). The shield of a nuclear reactor is a body of material surrounding the reactor to prevent the escape of neutrons and radiation into a protected area, which frequently is the entire space external to the reactor. It may be required for the safety of personnel or to reduce radiation enough to allow use of counting instruments for research or for locating contamination or airborne radioactivity.

Sievert: The new special unit of dose equivalent. The sievert equals the absorbed dose in gray times the quality factor for the radiation in question. (Symbol: Sv)

Specific Activity: Total activity of a given nuclide per gram of a compound, element, or radioactive nuclide.

Specific Gamma-Ray Constant: For a nuclide emitting gamma radiation, the product of exposure rate at a given distance from a point source of that nuclide and the square of that distance divided by the activity of the source, neglecting attenuation.

Spectrum: A visual display, a photographic record, or a plot of the distribution of the intensity of radiation of a given kind as a function of its wavelength, energy, frequency, momentum, mass, or any related quantity.

Standard, Radioactive: A sample of radioactive material, usually with a long half-life, in which the number and type of radioactive atoms at a definite reference time are known. It may be used as a radiation source for calibrating radiation measurement equipment.

Survey, Radiologic: Evaluation of the radiation hazards incident to the production, use, or existence of radioactive materials or other sources of radiation under specific conditions. Such evaluation customarily includes a physical survey of the disposition of materials and equipment, measurements or estimates of the levels of radiation that may be involved, and sufficient knowledge of processes using or affecting these materials to predict hazards resulting from expected or possible changes in materials or equipment.

Survey Meter (Laboratory Monitor): A detection instrument used to monitor an area for unsuspected radiation or to search for a lost radiation source or contamination.

T

Therapy: Medical treatment of a disease.

Brachytherapy (therapy at short distances): The treatment of disease with sealed radioactive sources placed near, or inserted directly into, the diseased area.

Contact Radiation Therapy: X-ray therapy with specially constructed tubes in which the target-skin distance is very short (less than 2 cm). The voltage is usually 40 to 60 kV.

Radiation Therapy: Treatment of disease with any type of radiation.

Rotation Therapy: Radiation therapy during which either the patient is rotated in front of the source of radiation or the source is revolved around the patient. In this way, a larger dose is built up at the center of rotation within the patient's body than on any area of the skin.

Teletherapy (therapy at long distance): The treatment of disease with gamma radiation at a distance from the patient.

Threshold, Photoelectric: The quantum of energy $h\nu_0$ that is just enough to release an electron from a given system in the photoelectric effect. The corresponding frequency, ν_0, and wavelength, λ_0, are the threshold frequency and wavelength respectively. For example, in the surface photoelectric effect, the threshold $h\nu_0$ for a particular surface is the energy of a photon which, when incident on the surface, causes the electron to emerge with zero kinetic energy.

Tissue Equivalent Material: Material made up of the same elements in the same proportions as they occur in a particular biologic tissue. In some cases, the equivalence may be approximated with sufficient accuracy on the basis of effective atomic number.

Townsend Avalanche: (See Avalanche.)

U

Umbra: The region within the beam receiving the full strength of the primary x- or gamma-ray photons.

Uncontrolled Area: An area not under the authority of the Radiation Protection Officer and not subject to restriction due to the presence of radiation.

V

Valence: Number representing the combining or displacing power of an atom; number of electrons lost, gained, or shared by an atom in a compound; number of hydrogen atoms with which an atom will combine, or which it will displace.

Volt: The unit of electromotive force ($1V = 1JC^{-1}$).

Voltage: The potential difference, in volts, between two different points in an electric circuit or between two different electrodes.

Voltage, Operating: As applied to radiation detection instruments, the voltage across the electrodes in the detecting chamber required for proper detection of an ionizing event.

Voltage, Starting: For a counter tube, the minimum voltage that must be applied to obtain counts with the particular circuit with which it is associated.

Volume, Sensitive: That portion of a counter tube or ionization chamber which responds to a specific radiation.

W

Watt: The unit of power equal to 1 joule per second ($1W = 1\ J\ s^{-1}$).

Wavelength: Distance between any two similar points of two consecutive waves (λ) for electromagnetic radiation. The wavelength is equal to the velocity of light (c) divided by the frequency of the wave (ν), $\lambda = c/\nu$. The "effective wavelength" is the wavelength of monochromatic x-rays that would undergo the same percentage attenuation in a specified filter as the heterogeneous beam under consideration.

Wave Motion: The transmission of a periodic motion or vibration through a medium or empty space. *Transverse*: Wave motion in which the vibration is perpendicular to the direction of propagation. *Longitudinal*: Wave motion in which the vibration is parallel to the direction of propagation.

X

X-Rays: Penetrating electromagnetic radiations whose wavelengths are shorter than those of visible light. They are usually produced by bombarding a metallic target with fast electrons in a high vacuum. In nuclear reactions, it is customary to refer to photons originating in the nucleus as gamma-rays, and those originating in the extranuclear part of the atom as x-rays. These rays are sometimes called roentgen rays after their discoverer, W.C. Roentgen.

INDEX

Page numbers in *italics* indicate illustrations; page numbers followed by t indicate tables.

Index